Praise for *The Out-of-Sync Child*

"This book is grea _____ ents of the many children wh _____ et parents off the hook of bla _____ hem get on to the job of addres _____ ies."

—T. Berr _____ hpoints Center,
Boston Children's Hospital

"Once again, Carol brings her warmth, wisdom, and compassion to families, teachers, and others yearning to understand and manage sensory processing difficulties. This fresh and lively updated edition brings you even more insights and advice you can use to help your child, student, or even yourself to play more, learn more, and thrive to the utmost."

—Lindsey Biel, MA, OTR/L, coauthor of *Raising a Sensory Smart Child*

"Carol Stock Kranowitz has helped many parents understand more about [sensory processing disorder] and how it manifests itself in children."

—*Sunday News* (Lancaster, PA)

"Kranowitz writes intelligently about a bewildering topic. . . . In concise, well-organized chapters, Kranowitz reveals how the tactile, vestibular (pertaining to gravity and movement), and proprioceptive (pertaining to joints, muscles, and ligaments) senses operate. . . . [She] helps clear the way for families to understand a disorder that they may suspect but have not been able to pinpoint."

—*Publishers Weekly*

"A book that demystifies [sensory processing disorder]. As a music, movement, and drama teacher, [Kranowitz] has developed a purposeful curriculum that integrates sensorimotor activities into the pre-school day."

—*The Ithaca Journal* (Ithaca, NY)

"Warm and wise, this book will bring both hope and practical help to parents who wonder why their kid doesn't 'fit in.'"

—Jane M. Healy, PhD, learning specialist and author of
Your Child's Growing Mind

"*The Out-of-Sync Child* does a masterful job of describing the different ways children react to sensations and integrate their responses to their world. The book provides detailed, practical information that will help parents understand how the nervous system works."

—Stanley I. Greenspan, MD, child psychiatrist and author (with Serena Wieder) of *The Child with Special Needs*

"Comprehensive yet easy to understand . . . helpful tools for parents to promote healthy integration.

"*The Out-of-Sync Child* is written for and can be easily understood by parents and non-professionals. Carol Stock Kranowitz's description and discussion of [sensory processing disorder] give a clear and concise picture of a disability. This book is a model for taking a little-known and often-missed disability and making it accessible to the people most in need of this information.

"Kranowitz gives excellent examples of typical indicators that can signal a parent (or caregiver) that a [sensory processing disorder] may be present. . . . [She also] gives the reader concrete information and a testing checklist to help evaluate whether a child might have a [sensory processing disorder].

"This is a great book and a must-read for any parent who thinks their child might have unusual behavior difficulties. Kranowitz avoids hypertechnical language and explanations. Instead, her treatment of sensory integration issues relies on common sense and clear examples. The book is so well written that readers will be tempted to use Kranowitz's analytical approach when they read about other behavior or learning disabilities. Its calming tone and no-nonsense approach give parents the power to positively address their child's [sensory processing disorder]."

—*The Exceptional Parent*

The Out-of-Sync Child

The
Out-of-Sync
Child

Recognizing and Coping with
Sensory Processing Differences

THIRD EDITION (2022)

Carol Stock Kranowitz, M.A.

A TarcherPerigee Book

tarcherperigee

an imprint of Penguin Random House LLC
penguinrandomhouse.com

Originally published in a different form in 1998 and 2006, by Perigee,
an imprint of The Berkley Publishing Group, a division of
Penguin Random House, LLC.

Most TarcherPerigee books are available at special quantity discounts for bulk
purchase for sales promotions, premiums, fund-raising, and educational needs.
Special books or book excerpts also can be created to fit specific needs. For
details, write: SpecialMarkets@penguinrandomhouse.com.

Third edition ISBN: 9780593419410

PUBLISHING HISTORY
Original Perigee trade paperback edition / March 1998
Revised Perigee trade paperback edition / August 2006
TarcherPerigee trade paperback edition / April 2022

Printed in the United States of America
5th Printing

Book design by Patrice Sheridan

Contents

PART 1

Recognizing Sensory Processing Differences

PART 2

Coping with
Sensory Processing Differences

Foreword to the Third Edition

In 1955, A. Jean Ayres, PhD, wrote her first article related to the theory of sensory integration; in 1972, her first book was published, and an entire field was launched. Based on her work, Carol Kranowitz, a preschool educator, helped dozens of children who manifested "sensory integration (SI) dysfunction" with the consultation of an occupational therapist (OT) who had studied Dr. Ayres's work. Dr. Ayres died in 1988, and with her went the knowledge base and energy that only a founder of a new vision can have. Although OTs still practiced and taught courses on SI, the field had lost its leader.

In 1998, Carol published *The Out-of-Sync Child,* written for parents and teachers. The book was a down-to-earth explanation of: 1) the complex theory of sensory integration; 2) the treatment, occupational therapy with a sensory integration approach (OT-SI); and 3) the disorder, now called sensory processing disorder (SPD). Her book reenergized the world of SI. Clutching it in their hands, parents came into pediatricians' and OTs' clinics, saying, "This is my child. We need occupational therapy."

Carol's goal was to write a guidebook for parents whose children had sensory processing issues. The popularity of this best seller demonstrates both her success in achieving that goal and the urgent need for a book of this sort. *The Out-of-Sync Child* helps parents discover the missing sensory piece in their kid's puzzle. Relieved, they see that their child's disturbing behaviors or disorganized motor abilities are related to SPD; as one parent put it, "The problem is physical, not parental."

Parents ask, "How could my child's problem have been overlooked for so long?" The answer is that few professionals, outside of OTs, knew about SPD. When Carol's book took off, the picture changed. *The Out-of-Sync Child* is on every special needs reading list and in the curriculum of many educational programs. It is the first book that OTs hand to bewildered, frustrated parents when they come to a clinic for answers.

Now we have the third edition, with updated definitions, more information about "look-alike" conditions and children with autism, and a refreshed look at diagnosis and treatment. The explanations of differences in sensory modulation, sensory discrimination, and sensory-based motor abilities provide needed clarification of SPD's subtypes. In her goal to write for nonscientists, Carol has succeeded again!

In this decade, I predict that we will see more scientific publications on SPD, its inclusion in standard diagnostic manuals, and more children getting a correct diagnosis and appropriate treatment. We will witness a generation of children with sensory processing differences growing competent and successful at home and school. We will see OT-SI accepted by mainstream medical and educational professionals.

Carol's contribution to the field has been immeasurable. With her book came understanding and hope where none had been before for thousands of parents. Hope . . . and action . . . and children with brighter futures and more fulfilled lives. What could be more valuable?

Lucy Jane Miller, PhD, OTR, FAOTA
Founder Emeritus, STAR Institute for Sensory Processing
Author, *Sensational Kids: Hope and Help for Children with Sensory Processing Disorder*

Acknowledgments

Primarily, I am profoundly grateful to the late A. Jean Ayres, PhD, OTR, whom I never met but shall revere forever. Her work has touched and moved me to do all I can for children with sensory processing differences—and for their grown-ups.

I also thank all those who made the first edition of this book possible:

Occupational therapists Lynn A. Balzer-Martin, Georgia deGangi, Sheri Present, Susanne Smith Roley, and Trude Turnquist.

Child development specialists and advocates T. Berry Brazelton, Michael Castleberry, Stanley Greenspan, Jane Healy, Anne Kendall, Patricia Lemer, Larry Silver, and Karen Strimple.

Parents Chris Bridgeman, Catherine and Ron Butler, Deborah Thommasen, Linda Finkel and Vivek Talvadkar, Jacquie and Paul London, Mary Eager, and Denise McMillen.

Teachers and students at St. Columba's Nursery School in Washington, DC; Lynn Sonberg and Meg Schneider of Skylight; Sheila Curry Oakes, my first Perigee editor; T. J. Wylie, illustrator; and my peerless family.

For this third edition, my everlasting love and thanks go to Lucy Jane Miller, PhD, who has gently guided my thinking and raised my level of understanding about sensory processing. Additionally, I thank these marvelous professionals for their wisdom and support throughout the years:

Occupational therapists Paula Aquilla, Kelly Beins, June Bunch, Anita Bundy, Sharon Cermak, Robyn Chu, Valerie Dejean, Winnie Dunn, Kimberly Geary, Jill Guz, Barbara Hanft, Diana Henry, Jan Hollenbeck, Genevieve Jereb, Nancy Kashman, Lorna Jean King, Moya Kinnealey, Jane Koomar, Cara Koscinski, Aubrey Lande, Shelly Lane, Barbara Lindner, Teresa May-Benson, Heather Miller-Kuhaneck, Maura Mooneyham, Myania Moses, Mim Ochsenbein, Lisa Porter, Sherry Shellenberger, Sarah Schoen, Virginia Spielmann, Janet Stafford, Stacey Szklut, Sandy Wainman, Rondalyn Whitney, Sue Wilkinson, Mary Sue Williams, and so many more.

Developmental optometrists Sanford Cohen and Charles Shidlofsky; developmental pediatrician Dan Shapiro; nutritionist Kelly Dorfman; pediatric neurologist Elysa Marco; perceptual-motor therapist Joye Newman; reading specialist Debra Em Wilson; special needs care navigator Sarah Wayland; speech-language pathologists Laura Glaser, Janet Mora, and Kathleen Morris; 2e specialist Julie Skolnick; and other influential individuals, including Julia Berry, David Brown, Laurie Friedman, Temple Grandin, Laurie Renke, Rachel Schneider, Stephen Shore, Mark Zweig, and my devoted editor at TarcherPerigee, Marian Lizzi.

I remain eternally in your debt.

Carol Stock Kranowitz
Bethesda, Maryland
Spring 2022

Introduction

For twenty-five years, I taught at St. Columba's Nursery School in Washington, DC. Most preschoolers loved my classes involving music, movement, and dramatic play. Every day, small groups of three-, four-, and five-year-olds would come to my room to play, move, and learn. They happily pounded on drums and xylophones, sang and clapped, danced and twirled. They shook beanbags, manipulated puppets, and enacted fairy tales. They waved the parachute, played musical follow-the-leader games, and flowed through obstacle courses. They swooped like kites, stomped like elephants, and melted like snowmen.

Most children enjoy such activities because they have effective sensory processing—the ability to organize sensory information for use in daily life. They take in the sensations of touch, movement, sight, and sound coming from their bodies and the world around them, and they respond in a well-regulated way.

Some children, however, such as Andrew, Ben, and Alice, did not enjoy coming to my classroom. Faced with the challenge of sensory-motor experiences, they became tense, unhappy, and confused. They refused to participate in the activities, or did so ineffectively, and their behavior disrupted their classmates' fun. They are the children for whom this book is written.

In my teaching career (1976–2001), I worked with more

than one thousand young children. Outside of school, I taught music classes for kindergartners in my home. I choreographed children's dances for community performances. I conducted dozens of musical birthday parties. I was room mother, Cub Scout den leader, and team manager for my own sons' school and sports groups.

Many years of working with children taught me that *all* children like lively, interesting activities. They all want to join the fun—yet some do not take part. Why not? Is it that they *won't*—or that they *can't*?

When I began teaching, the nonparticipants puzzled me. Why, I wondered, were these children so difficult to reach? Why did they fall apart when it was time to join the fun?

Why did Andrew buzz around the room's perimeter while his classmates, sitting on the rug, sang "The Wheels on the Bus"?

Why did Ben tap, tap, tap his shoulders when the musical instructions were to tap, tap, tap his knees?

Why did Alice flop onto her stomach, "too tired" to sit up and strike together two rhythm sticks?

At first, these children annoyed me. They made me feel like a bad teacher. They also made me feel like a bad person when their inattention or disruptive behavior caused me to react negatively. Indeed, on one regrettable occasion, I told a child that turning away and covering his ears when I played the guitar was "just plain rude." That day I went home and wept.

Every evening, while preparing dinner or engaging with my sons, I would muse about these students. I could not get a handle on them. They had no identified special needs. They weren't unloved or disadvantaged. Some seemed to misbehave on purpose, like sticking a foot out to trip a classmate, while others seemed to move without any purpose at all, in an aimless or listless manner. Little about their behavior could be classified except for a shared inability to enjoy the activities that children traditionally relish.

I wasn't the only one who was stumped. Karen Strimple, director of St. Columba's Nursery School, and the other teachers were equally puzzled by the same children. The children's parents were often concerned, especially when they compared their child's behavior with that of their other, more "together" offspring. And if caring parents and teachers were frustrated, how must the children themselves feel?

They felt like failures.

And we teachers felt that we were failing them.

We knew we could do better. After all, since the 1970s, St. Columba's had been mainstreaming into its regular school program a number of children with identified special needs. We were extremely successful with these children. Why were we less successful teaching certain "regular" kids with subtle, unidentified problems? We wanted an answer.

The answer came from Lynn A. Balzer-Martin, PhD, a St. Columba parent and a pediatric occupational therapist. Since the 1970s, Lynn had been an educational consultant for our mainstreaming program—called inclusion today. Her primary work, however, was diagnosing and treating young children who had academic and behavior problems stemming from a neurological inefficiency—then called "sensory integration dysfunction."

An occupational therapist, A. Jean Ayres, PhD, was the pioneer who first described the problem. In the mid-twentieth century, Dr. Ayres formulated a theory of sensory integration dysfunction and led other occupational therapists in developing intervention strategies. Her book *Sensory Integration and the Child* presents a thorough explanation of this misunderstood problem and is required reading for anyone interested in grasping its technicalities.

Sensory integration dysfunction (sensory processing disorder or sensory processing differences) is not a new problem. It is a new definition of an old problem.

Sensory processing differences (SPD) can cause a bewildering variety of symptoms. When their central nervous systems are ineffective in processing sensory information, children have a hard time functioning in daily life. They may look fine and have superior intelligence but may be awkward and clumsy, fearful and withdrawn, or hostile and aggressive. SPD can affect not only how they move and learn, but also how they behave, how they play and make friends, and especially how they feel about themselves.

Many parents, educators, doctors, and mental health professionals have difficulty recognizing SPD. When they do not recognize the problem, they may mistake a child's behavior, low self-esteem, or reluctance to participate in ordinary childhood experiences for hyperactivity, learning disabilities, or emotional problems. Unless they are educated about SPD, few people understand that bewildering behavior may stem from a poorly functioning nervous system.

Dr. Lynn Balzer-Martin, like other students of Dr. Ayres's work, was trained to recognize and treat sensory problems. Her growing concern was that many of her clients were not sent to her for a diagnosis until well after they had run into trouble at school or at home, at the ages of six, seven, or eight. She was anxious to identify children at younger ages because the brain is most receptive to change while it is developing.

Preschoolers, whose nervous systems are still developing

rapidly, stand a good chance to benefit from therapeutic intervention. Lynn knew that if SPD could be detected in three-, four-, or five-year-olds, these children could receive individualized treatment that would prevent later social and academic impasses.

The challenge was to find a way to identify preschoolers with SPD, because the available standardized tests are inappropriate for the "little guys." Lynn conceived of a quick, effective screening to see whether very young children had the neurological foundations necessary for developing into well-organized people. She asked us if we were interested.

Were we interested?!

Thus, everything came together at once. We wanted to learn more about our worrisome students. Lynn wanted to try out her screening idea. The Katharine P. Maddux Foundation, which already funded our flagship mainstreaming program, was urging us to develop more projects designed to improve the physical, mental, and emotional health of children and their families.

Lynn's first goal was to educate us about sensory processing and then, with our help, to devise a screening program that would be developmentally suitable for preschoolers.

The screening process would be fun for the children. It would be simple enough for many schools to duplicate. It would be short yet thorough enough to enable educators to distinguish between basic immaturity and possible SPD in young children.

Most important, it would provide data that would encourage parents to seek early intervention for their children with an appropriate professional (such as an occupational therapist, a physical therapist, or sometimes a psychologist or speech/language pathologist). The purpose of early intervention is to help children function better—even beautifully—in their class-rooms, in their homes, and in their daily lives.

In 1987, with the support of the school community and with my eager assistance, Lynn instituted a program at St. Columba's in which all 130 students undergo an annual screening.[1] We began to guide identified children into therapy. And we began to see immediate, positive, exhilarating results as these children's skills began to improve.

With Lynn's guidance, I studied and learned everything I could about the subject. I learned to screen the children and to compile data gleaned from teachers, parents, and direct observations. I learned to make sense of some children's mystifying behavior.

As my knowledge increased, so did my teaching skills. I learned to help my co-teachers understand why these children marched to a different drummer. I gave workshops at other pre-schools and elementary schools to train educators to recognize signs of this subtle problem. I added activities in my class that promoted healthy sensory-motor development for *all* children.

I rejoiced in the strides that children such as Andrew, Ben, and Alice made soon after they began occupational therapy. Incredibly, as they acquired more efficient sensory-motor skills, they relaxed, became more focused, and began to enjoy school. Now, when I went home at the end of the day, it wasn't to weep—it was to celebrate!

While my expertise grew, I learned that explaining SPD to parents requires time and skill. When children who were screened showed clear evidence of sensory processing differences, Karen and I asked their parents to come in to observe them in the classroom and on the playground. Then we would sit down for a private conference to discuss our observations.

In these conferences, we described what we observed to be their child's sensory processing difficulties. We explained that the problem was treatable. We said that while older children and even adults could improve with treatment, early intervention produced the most dramatic results. We tried to allay the parents' fears, assuring them that SPD did not suggest that their child was mentally deficient, or that they were inadequate parents.

We understood that this information inevitably filled parents with anxiety, questions, and misapprehensions. Often, they dashed to their pediatrician, who, unfamiliar with SPD, mistakenly dismissed it as a problem that the child would outgrow.

We knew that we raised more questions than it was possible to answer in a half-hour conference.

Thus, this book was conceived to explain sensory processing and its counterpart, SPD, to parents, teachers, and other non-OTs who were new at this. This third edition contains up-to-date information that may also help those who are already experienced in caring for children with other, more observable disabilities, many overlapping with SPD.

I have attempted to make the explanations reader-friendly. They will remind or introduce you to terms that child development professionals commonly use—terms with which you need to be familiar.

The viewpoint is "teacherly" and may differ here and there from a clinical or research-oriented point of view. Understanding SPD will allow you to understand your child (or student) better, and that is the book's most important purpose. Then you will be prepared to provide the help the child needs to become as competent and confident as possible.

How to Use This Book

Whether or not your child has been diagnosed, this book will help you understand and cope with sensory processing differences, which, when severe, are called sensory processing disorder (SPD). The book is not just for parents. It is also for teachers, medical doctors, occupational therapists, psychologists, grandparents, babysitters, and others who care for the out-of-sync child.

As a teacher, I have witnessed how SPD plays out. I have seen behavior that parents, pediatricians, and even therapists do not have the chance to observe. Thus, the book, written from a teacher's perspective, offers insights that a specialist in another field of child development might overlook.

Part 1 includes an introduction to four children with SPD; an overview of SPD and how it affects children's behavior; checklists (for you to mark) of symptoms and characteristics of out-of-sync children; associated problems and "look-alike" diagnoses; a guide to typical neurological development; how the fundamental senses work, how they influence everyday life, and what happens when they are inefficient; anecdotes contrasting the responses of children with and without efficient sensory processing; and the hope that a solution to your child's challenges is at hand.

Part 2 includes criteria and guidance for getting a diagnosis and treatment; examples of homemade charts for documenting your child's behavior; tips for keeping a running record; how occupational therapy helps, and a look at other therapies; suggestions for a sensory-enriched life and for improving your child's skills at home; ideas to share with teachers for helping your child at school; coping techniques to handle your child's emotions and to improve family life; and encouragement and advice—for you and your child are not alone!

The Out-of-Sync Child concludes with two appendixes: the sensory processing machine (to explain the role of the central nervous system) and Dr. Ayres's four levels of sensory integration, the notes, a glossary, and an index.

Read the book cover to cover to get a broad picture of SPD. Use it as a reference to refresh yourself on a specific area of sensory processing differences. With pencil in hand, use it as a workbook. Keep it handy as an activity book. Use it to learn about your child—and perhaps to learn about yourself as well.

A Word About Words
and That Pesky "D" in "SPD"

The acronym SPD is used throughout this book. "S" is for "Sensory." "P" is for "Processing." And "D" is for . . . Dysfunction? Disorder? Delays? Deficits? Disabilities? Difficulties? Dimensions? Diversity? Differences? Take your pick!

To explain . . .

The late A. Jean Ayres, PhD, an occupational therapist (abbreviated as OT), was the first to describe sensory problems as the result of inefficient neurological processing. In the mid-twentieth century, she developed a theory of sensory integration and taught other OTs how to assess "sensory integrative problems," which she also called "dysfunctions" and "disorders."[1]

Many brilliant OTs—Dr. Ayres's colleagues and disciples—continued her work. They used various terms, such as "sensory integration dysfunction" or "SI dysfunction." This mouthful was occasionally abbreviated to "SID," but that was a problem because SIDS is the acronym for sudden infant death syndrome. For a while, to avoid confusion, "DSI" was used, for "dysfunction in sensory integration." The American Occupational Therapy Association uses the term "sensory integration and processing challenges." Some practitioners prefer to call their intervention "Ayres sensory integration."[2]

In 1998, the first edition of this book was published. Its

subtitle is *Recognizing and Coping with Sensory Integration Dysfunction* because that was the term in use.

"Dysfunction," however, sounds negative. The fact that a child never lets his feet leave the ground or always is up to his armpits in mud does not mean that the child is abnormal or unhealthy.

For the child's sake, using consistent terminology is imperative so that OTs, doctors, other health professionals, parents, educators, and insurance companies can understand one another and agree on a diagnosis and its appropriate treatment. Thus, using Dr. Ayres's original concepts, a group led by Lucy Jane Miller, PhD, proposed to clarify the terminology.[3]

Their goal (partially met) was to have the condition acknowledged and included in the *Diagnostic and Statistical Manual of Mental Disorders, 5th Edition* (*DSM-5*), so that children with sensory processing differences could get an assessment and diagnosis. In their classification, sensory processing disorder is the overall term, encompassing three diagnostic groups—sensory modulation disorder, sensory discrimination disorder, and sensory-based motor disorder—and their subtypes.

In 2005, the second edition of this book was published. Its subtitle is *Recognizing and Coping with Sensory Processing Disorder* because that was the term in use.

"Disorder," however, is not the right word. Unless symptoms are found to impact the ability of an individual child or adult to function in daily life, atypical sensory processing is not considered a disorder. Disorders are signs of illness or dysfunctional health, such as anxiety, depression, and ADHD. For many children with sensory processing problems, the word "disorder" does not fit.

As scientific knowledge evolves, updated terms are being considered. Dr. Miller and colleagues are proposing the use of a dimensional approach. In an upcoming diagnostic tool, the Sensory Processing 3-Dimensions Scale (SP3D), they measure the presence of sensory differences along a continuum, ranging from mild to severe.[4]

In the right context, "dimensions" fits. So do other "D" words mentioned in the first paragraph.

In 2022, this third edition of the book has been published. Its subtitle is *Understanding and Coping with Sensory Processing Differences.* The term "differences" indicates that each person processes sensations in a unique way. Everyone can get in sync with that idea!

Throughout the book, I use the acronym SPD because it encompasses all of the "D's." Dear Reader: Please think of that pesky "D" as you like.

The

Out-of-Sync
Child

PART 1

Recognizing Sensory Processing Differences

1

Four Out-of-Sync Children at Home and School

NOTE: Mild sensory processing challenges are "differences." More pronounced challenges are "difficulties." Severe challenges are a "disorder." In this book, the "D" in the acronym SPD can stand for all three. (See "A Word About Words," page xxv.)

Surely you know a child who is oversensitive, clumsy, picky, fidgety, and out of sync. That child may be your son or daughter, your student or Scout, your nephew or neighbor . . . or the child you were, once upon a time.

That child may have sensory processing differences, difficulties, or disorder (SPD), a common, but misunderstood, problem that affects children's behavior, influencing the way they move, learn, communicate, relate to others, and feel about themselves. SPD can stand alone, or it can accompany other physical, cognitive, language, social, and emotional challenges.

To illustrate how SPD plays out, here are the stories of four out-of-sync children and the parents struggling to raise them. Perhaps you will recognize familiar signs in the child you know.

Whether sensory processing differences are major or minor,

the child who is out of sync needs understanding and support, for no child can overcome the obstacles alone.

Tommy

Tommy is the only son of two adoring parents. They waited a long time before having a child and rejoiced in his arrival. And when they finally got him in their hands, they got a handful.

The day after he was born, his wailing in the hospital nursery kept the other infants awake. Once he arrived home, he rarely slept through the night. Although he nursed well and grew rapidly, he adamantly rejected the introduction of solid food and vigorously resisted being weaned. He did not welcome cuddling; in fact, he seemed to hate it. He was a very fussy baby.

Today, Tommy is a fussy three-year-old. He is crying because his shoes are too tight, his socks too lumpy. He yanks them off and hurls them away.

To prevent a tantrum, his mother lets him wear bedroom slippers to school. She has learned that if it is not shoes and socks that bother him, it is inevitably something else that will trip him up during the day.

His parents bend over backward, but pleasing their healthy, attractive child is hard. Everything scares him or makes him miserable. His response to the world is "Oh, no!" He hates the playground, the beach, and the bathtub. He refuses to wear hats or mittens, even on the coldest days. Getting him to eat is a trial.

Arranging playdates with other children is a nightmare. Going to the barbershop is a disaster. Wherever they go, people turn away—or stare.

His teacher reports that he avoids painting and other messy activities. He fidgets at story time and does not pay attention.

He lashes out at his classmates for no apparent reason. He is, however, the world's best block-builder, as long as he is not crowded.

Tommy's pediatrician tells his parents nothing is wrong with him, so they should stop worrying and just let him grow. His grandparents say he's spoiled and needs stricter discipline. Friends suggest going on a vacation without him.

Tommy's parents wonder if yielding to his whims is wise, but it is the only method that works. They are exhausted, frustrated, and stressed. They cannot understand why he is so different from other children.

Vicki

Sweet Vicki, a pudgy first-grader, is often in a daze. Her response to the world buzzing around her seems to be "Wait, what?" She does not seem to see where she is going, so she bumps into furniture and stumbles on grass. When she tumbles, she is slow to extend her foot or hand to break the fall. She does not appear to hear ordinary sounds, either. Other six-year-olds may have developed the sense to stop, look, and listen, but Vicki is different. She needs a lot more sensory input than they do to catch on and catch up.

In addition, Vicki fatigues easily. A family outing or a trip to the playground quickly wears her out. She says with a sigh, "You go. I don't want to. I'm too pooped."

Because of her lethargy, her parents find that getting her out of bed, asking her to put on her coat, or maneuvering her into the car is an ordeal. She takes a long time to carry out simple, familiar movements. In every situation, it is as if she is saying, "What does that sensation mean? How am I supposed to use it?"

Nonetheless, she wants to be a ballerina when she grows up. Every day she sprawls in front of the TV to watch her favorite video, *The Nutcracker*. When her beloved Sugar Plum Fairies begin to dance, she hauls herself up to sway along with them. Her movements, however, do not match the musical rhythm or tempo. Ear-body coordination is not her forte.

Vicki begged for ballet lessons, but they have not been going well. She loves her purple tutu but cannot differentiate top from bottom and needs help to get into it. Once attired in tulle, tiara, and slippers, she plops down. She has no idea how to bend her knees in a plié or stretch her leg in an arabesque. At dancing school, Vicki usually gets cold feet and clings like taffy to her mother's leg.

Vicki's parents disagree on the best way to handle her. Her father picks her up and puts her places—in bed, in the car, on a chair. He also dresses her, as she has trouble orienting her limbs to get into her clothes. He refers to her as his "little noodle."

Vicki's mother, on the other hand, believes Vicki will never learn to move with confidence, much less become a ballerina, if she does not learn independence. Her mother says, "I think she would stick to one spot all day if I let her."

Although Vicki lacks "oomph" and is definitely not a self-starter, certain kinds of movement will get her on her toes. She becomes livelier after getting into unusual positions—rocking forward and backward while on all fours, hanging over the edge of her bed upside-down, and swinging on her tummy. While she cannot yet pump, she loves to be pushed on the playground swing for a long time—and when she stops, she is never dizzy, as other children might be.

Being pushed *passively* arouses Vicki, as does *actively* pushing something heavy. Occasionally, she crams books into her doll carriage and shoves it around the house. She volunteers to push the grocery cart and carry bags into the house. She also enjoys pulling her big sister in a wagon. After pushing and pulling weighty loads, she has some energy for half an hour or so and then sinks back into her customary lethargy.

At school, Vicki mostly sits. Her teacher says, "Vicki has difficulty socializing and getting involved in classroom activities. It's like her batteries are low. She needs a jump start just to get going. Then she loses interest and gives up easily."

Vicki's behavior mystifies her parents. Their experiences with their two other active children have not prepared them to deal with her differences.

Paul

Paul is an extremely shy ten-year-old. He moves awkwardly, has poor posture and balance, and falls frequently. He lacks the know-how to play, and when he's in a group with other children, he usually watches dolefully or shuffles away. At their grandparents' house one Sunday afternoon, Paul's twelve-year-old cousin, Prescott, invites Paul to play marbles and shoot baskets with him. Paul gives the activities a halfhearted try, shrugs, and turns away. "I can't do that," he says. "Anyway, what's the point?"

Paul dislikes school. Sometimes he asks to stay home and his parents let him. He says he does not want to go to school because he's different from all the other kids. He says he is no good at anything, and everyone laughs at him.

Paul's teacher notes that he has a long attention span and an above-average reading ability. She wonders why a child with so much information to share becomes paralyzed when he has to write a paper. True, his handwriting is laborious, and his papers are crumpled and full of erasure holes. True, he has a "death grip" on pencils, fixes his elbow to his ribs, and sticks his tongue out when he writes. True, he often slips off the chair when he is concentrating hard on written work. His handwriting skills, she hopes, will improve with more practice. She says he just needs to get organized so that he can pay more attention to his assignments and do neater work.

His parents wonder why he is a misfit at school, because he has always fit right into their sedate lifestyle. Paul is a modest child, rarely seeking attention. He can spend hours slumped over his baseball cards, completely self-absorbed.

Paul's parents think he is the perfect child. They observe that he is different from other kids, who are loud and mischievous. He never makes trouble, although he is somewhat clumsy, often dropping dishes and breaking toys that require simple manipulation. But then his parents are somewhat clumsy, too, and have come to believe that physical prowess is unimportant. They are glad that their son is quiet, well-mannered, and bookish, just like them.

Something, however, is getting in his way. His parents have no idea what.

Sebastian

Sebastian, eight, fidgets constantly. At school, he riffles book pages, twiddles with markers, taps rulers, and snaps pencils. He clicks his teeth and chews his collar.

Sebastian's eyes dart, knees bounce, feet tap, and fingers flap his earlobes. He tips his desk chair way back and then brings it forward with a jolt. He squirms in his seat, sitting on his feet or squeezing his knees to his chest. He jumps out of his seat every chance he gets to sharpen his pencil or pitch a wadded paper toward the wastebasket.

His nonstop activity distracts his classmates and teacher. He used to twirl the lanyard with his latchkey around his finger. Once he let go accidentally and it whirled across the room and hit the window. Now he hands the lanyard over to his teacher every morning so it won't annoy or hurt anyone.

Every child seeks sensory stimulation, but Sebastian's craving for sensations is different. "More, more, more!" He is the child who has "gotta touch" and "gotta move," even when it should be clear that touching and moving at that moment is inappropriate.

One day the teacher is preparing a science lesson. She lays out white glue, laundry borax, and water—the ingredients to make a pliable substance called "stretchy gook." Sebastian is interested and hovers nearby, twitching his fingers and hopping from foot to foot. The teacher says, "Please don't touch a thing until the other kids join us," but he reaches forward and knocks over the bottle of glue, spilling it across the table.

"Sebastian! You did it again!" the teacher says.

"I didn't mean to!" Sebastian cries. He shakes his head vigorously and jumps up and down. "Oh," he moans, "why do I always get in trouble?"

"Oh," moans the teacher, mopping up the mess, "what shall I do with you?"

Why are Tommy, Vicki, Paul, and Sebastian out of sync? Their parents, teachers, and pediatricians do not know what to think.

The children have no identified disabilities, such as autism, cerebral palsy, or impaired eyesight. They seem to have everything going for them: they are healthy, intelligent, and dearly loved. Yet they struggle with the basic skills of managing their responses to ordinary sensations, of planning and organizing their actions, and of regulating their attention and activity levels.

Their common problem is SPD.

2

Does Your Child Have Sensory Processing Differences?

Written in layperson's terms, this chapter about common symptoms and associated problems may help you determine whether SPD affects your child. If your child's sensory differences are obvious, the information may strike you like a bolt of lightning. You may instantly recognize the signs and be relieved to have some answers at last. Even if the differences are mild, you can use this information to gain new insight into your child's puzzling behavior.

SPD: A Brief Definition

SPD is a problem in receiving, integrating (i.e., connecting), interpreting, or using the information from one's senses to function smoothly in daily life. (Regarding the acronym SPD, see "A Word About Words," page xxv.)

The late A. Jean Ayres, PhD, an occupational therapist (OT), was the first to describe sensory processing difficulties as the result of differences in the central nervous system. In the mid-twentieth century, she developed a theory of sensory integration and taught other OTs how to assess it.

When mild, SPD can cause delays in developmental milestones, such as learning to walk later than most children. When severe, it can significantly hinder the development of self-regulation, movement, learning, language, and social/emotional skills. SPD may begin in utero, becoming evident in infancy, childhood, adolescence, or adulthood and usually lasting throughout a person's life span.

The chart shows three diagnostic groups and subtypes, based on terminology proposed by Lucy Jane Miller, PhD, a mentee of Dr. Ayres, and other esteemed OTs.[1] (Terms will be explained in chapter 4.)

SUBTYPES OF SPD

1. Sensory Modulation Differences			2. Sensory Discrimination Differences	3. Sensory-Based Motor Differences	
A. Sensory over-responsivity	B. Sensory under-responsivity	C. Sensory craving	Touch Movement Body position Sight Sound Smell Taste Internal organs	A. Postural challenges	B. Dyspraxia (movement and coordination problems)

Sensory processing happens in the central nervous system (CNS), at the "head" of which is the brain. When processing is inefficient in the brain, the child may be unable to perceive, register, or respond to sensory information to behave in a meaningful, consistent way. He may have difficulty using sensory information to plan and carry out actions that he needs to do. Thus, he may not learn easily.

Learning is a broad term. One kind of learning is called adaptive behavior, which is the ability to change one's behavior in response to new circumstances, such as learning to meet different teachers' expectations. Adaptive behavior (or adaptive responses) is goal-directed and purposeful.

Another kind of learning is motor learning, which is the ability to develop increasingly complex movement skills after one has mastered simpler ones. Examples are learning to use a pencil after learning to use a crayon, or learning to catch a ball after learning to throw one.

A third kind of learning is academic learning, or cognition. This is the ability to acquire conceptual skills, such as reading, computing, and applying what one learns today to what one learned yesterday.

The brain-behavior connection is very strong. Because the child with SPD has a disorganized brain, many aspects of his behavior are disorganized. His overall development is irregular, and his participation in childhood experiences is spotty, reluctant, or inept. For the out-of-sync child, performing ordinary tasks and responding to everyday events can be enormously challenging.

The inability to get through the day smoothly is not because the child won't, but because he can't.

How Inefficient Sensory Processing Leads to Inefficient Learning

Your child yanks the cat's tail and the cat hisses, arches its back, and spits. Normally, through experience, a child will learn not to repeat such a scary experience. He learns to be cautious. In the future, his behavior will be more adaptive.

The child with SPD, however, may have difficulty "reading cues," verbal or nonverbal, from the environment. He may not decode the auditory message of the cat's hostile hissing, the visual message of the cat's arched back, or the tactile message of spit on his cheek. He misses the "big picture" and may not learn appropriate caution.

Or the child can read the cat's reaction, but is unable to change his behavior and stop himself. He receives the sensory information, but cannot organize it to produce an efficient response.

Or the child sometimes can take in sensations, organize them, and respond appropriately—but not today. This may be one of his "off" days.

Possible results:

* The child may never learn and may get repeatedly scratched. Thus, he may continue this risky behavior until someone removes the cat, or the cat learns to avoid the child. The child loses a chance to learn how to relate positively to other living creatures.
* The child becomes fearful of the cat. He may not understand cause and effect and may be bewildered by what seems to be unpredictable cat behavior. He may become afraid of other animals, too.
* Eventually, the child may learn about cause and effect, may learn to grade his movements, may learn to treat animals gently, and may grow up to love cats—but this will happen only with much conscious effort, after much time and many, many scratches.

Common Symptoms of SPD

SPD has three subtypes. Below are checklists of these subtypes' common symptoms.

The first list, "Sensory Modulation Differences," pertains to how a child's brain reacts to sensations and regulates his responses. Some children with modulation differences are overresponsive. Overwhelmed by ordinary sensations, these extremely sensitive "sensory avoiders" cringe or appear resistant, crying, "Oh, no!" Some children are underresponsive; these "sensory stragglers" seem not to take in sensations, saying, "Wait, what?" Some children are sensory craving; these "sensory cravers" have an insatiable need for certain stimuli, calling, "More, more!"

Unofficial Terms to Describe Children with SPD

The terms in the first column are unscientific suggestions to help you picture children with different types of SPD.

This child:	Has difficulties due to:
Sensory Avoider	Overresponsivity
Sensory Straggler	Underresponsivity
Sensory Craver	Sensory craving
Sensory Jumbler	Discrimination differences
Sensory Slumper	Postural differences
Sensory Fumbler	Dyspraxia (poor coordination)

The second list, "Sensory Discrimination Differences," refers to challenges in distinguishing details of incoming messages within one sense. When sensory messages confuse a "sensory jumbler," her response is, "What does that sensory message mean?"

The third list, "Sensory-Based Motor Differences," concerns difficulties in using one's integrated senses to sit, move, write, eat, etc. One type of child, the "sensory slumper," has postural challenges, making it difficult to move and support his body during activities, saying, "Don't want to." Another type, the "sensory fumbler," struggles to come up with creative ideas, to make a "motor plan," and to carry out multistep actions, avowing, "I can't do that."

As you check the symptoms that you recognize, please understand that they will vary from child to child, because every brain, like every fingerprint or snowflake, is unique. No child will exhibit all the symptoms. Still, if several descriptions fit your son or daughter, chances are that he or she needs understanding and support. Ignoring these challenging differences will not make them disappear.

SENSORY MODULATION DIFFERENCES

The most common category of SPD is sensory modulation differences, seen when the sensory avoider, sensory straggler, or sensory craver exhibits one or more symptoms with frequency, intensity, and duration. Frequency means several times a day. Intensity means the magnitude of the experience; e.g., the child markedly keeps from—or leaps for—sensory stimuli. Duration means that the response lasts several minutes or hours.

These charts will give you a quick overview of common problems. Later chapters will provide more details.

While differences with touch, movement, and body position are the telltale signs of SPD, the child may also respond in atypical ways to sight, sound, smell, taste, and visceral input from internal organs:

Sensations	Sensory Avoider (Overresponsivity): "Oh, no!"	Sensory Straggler (Underresponsivity): "Wait, what?"	Sensory Craver (Craving): "More!"
Touch	☐ Avoids touching or being touched by objects and people. Reacts with a fight-or-flight response to getting dirty, to certain textures of clothing and food, and to light, unexpected touch.	☐ Is unaware of messy face, hands, or clothes, and may not know whether she has been touched. Does not notice how things feel and often drops items. Seems to lack "inner drive" to handle toys, utensils, pencils, tools.	☐ Constantly touches everything, wallows in mud, dumps out bins of toys and rummages through them purposelessly, and rubs against walls and furniture.
Movement and Balance	☐ Avoids moving or being unexpect-edly moved. Is insecure and anxious about falling or being off balance. Keeps feet on the ground. Gets carsick.	☐ Does not notice or object to being moved. Is unaware of falling and protects self poorly. Not a self-starter, but once started, swings for a long time without getting dizzy.	☐ Craves fast and spinning movement, and may not get dizzy. Moves constantly, fidgets, gets upside down, rocks on feet, is a daredevil, and takes bold risks.
Body Position and Muscle Control	☐ May avoid playground and sports activities.	☐ Seems to lack motivation to move. Sits in W position. While walking, slaps feet on ground for input. Becomes more alert after activity.	☐ Craves bear hugs and deep pressure. Constantly bumps and crashes, gnaws and chews. Seeks heavy work and vigorous movement.

Sensations	Sensory Avoider (Overresponsivity): "Oh, no!"	Sensory Straggler (Underresponsivity): "Wait, what?"	Sensory Craver (Craving): "More!"
Sight	☐ Gets overexcited with too much to look at (words, toys, or crowds). Covers eyes, has poor eye contact, is inattentive to desk work, overreacts to bright light. Is ever alert and watchful.	☐ Ignores novel visual stimuli, e.g., obstacles in path. Responds slowly to gestures or approaching objects. May not turn from bright light. Stares at and seems to look through faces and objects.	☐ Craves visually stimulating scenes and screens for lengthy times. Is attracted to shiny, spinning objects and bright, flickering strobe lights or sunlight streaming through blinds.
Sound	☐ Covers ears to close out sounds or voices. Complains about noises, such as vacuum cleaners or people singing, that do not bother others.	☐ Ignores ordinary sounds and voices, but may "turn on" to strong musical beats or extremely loud, close, or sudden sounds.	☐ Welcomes loud noises and TV volume. Loves crowds and places with noisy action. May speak in a booming voice.
Smell	☐ Objects to odors, e.g., perfume or food, that others like or do not notice.	☐ May be unaware of unpleasant odors and unable to smell his meal.	☐ Seeks strong odors, even objectionable ones, and sniffs food, people, and objects.

Sensations	Sensory Avoider (Overresponsivity): "Oh, no!"	Sensory Straggler (Underresponsivity): "Wait, what?"	Sensory Craver (Craving): "More!"
Taste	☐ Strongly objects to certain textures and temperatures of foods. May frequently gag while eating.	☐ May be able to eat very spicy food without complaint. Adds salt or spice to food to taste it.	☐ May lick or taste inedible objects, like Play-Doh and toys. May prefer very spicy or very hot foods.
Internal feelings	☐ Complains about heat, cold, thirst, and hunger. May have frequent stomachaches. Remembers past aches and pains such as splinters. May need to urinate often.	☐ May not notice thirst, hunger, upset stomach, pain, or emotions. May wet bed or pants, unaware of the need to urinate.	☐ May eat an entire pizza or gallon of ice cream and still want more.

SENSORY DISCRIMINATION DIFFERENCES

Another category pertains to sensory discrimination of the qualities of sensations within a sensory system. The child who easily discriminates a nickel from a dime by touch alone has an advantageous difference. The sensory jumbler who cannot discriminate the sound of "big" from "pig" has a disadvantageous difference. Often, he also has sensory-based motor and sensory modulation challenges.

Sensations	Sensory Jumbler (Discrimination Differences): "What does that mean?"
Touch	☐ Cannot tell where on her body she has been touched. Has poor body awareness; "out of touch" with hands and feet. Cannot distinguish objects by feel alone (without seeing). Is a sloppy dresser and very awkward with buttons, barrettes, etc. Handles eating utensils and classroom tools inefficiently. May have difficulty processing sensations of pain and temperature, e.g., gauging how serious a bruise is, or whether the room is overheated or chilly.
Movement and Balance	☐ Cannot feel himself falling, especially when eyes are closed. Becomes easily confused when turning, changing directions, or getting into a stance where his head is outside an upright, two-footed position. May be unable to tell when he has had enough movement.
Body Position and Muscle Control	☐ May be unfamiliar with own body. Is "klutzy" and has difficulty positioning limbs for getting dressed or pedaling a bike. Cannot grade (adjust) movements smoothly, using too much or not enough force for handling pencils and toys, or for pushing open doors and kicking balls. May bump, crash, and "dive-bomb" into others in interactions.

Sensations	Sensory Jumbler (Discrimination Differences): "What does that mean?"
Sight	☐ If problem is caused by SPD (and not nearsightedness, for example), may confuse likenesses and differences in pictures, written words, objects, and faces. In social interactions, may miss people's expressions and gestures. Has difficulty with visual tasks, such as lining up columns of numbers or judging where things are in space—himself included—and how to move to avoid bumping into objects.
Sound	☐ If problem is caused by SPD (and not ear infections or dyslexia, for example), may have difficulty recognizing the differences between sounds, especially consonants at ends of words. Cannot repeat or make up rhymes. Sings out of tune. Looks to others for cues, as verbal instructions may be confusing. Has poor auditory skills, such as picking out a teacher's voice from a noisy background, or paying attention to one sound without being distracted by other sounds.
Smell and Taste	☐ Cannot distinguish distinct smells such as lemons, vinegar, or soap. Cannot distinguish tastes or tell when food is too spicy, salty, or sweet. May choose or reject food based on the way it looks.

Sensations	Sensory Jumbler (Discrimination Differences): "What does that mean?"
Internal Feelings	□ May feel faint but not recognize that she is hungry. May feel discomfort but not realize she needs to have a bowel movement. May not know where her body aches or whether she feels hot or cold.

SENSORY-BASED MOTOR DIFFERENCES

The third SPD category is sensory-based motor differences, with two types. One type involves postural challenges with movement patterns, balance, and using both sides of the body together (bilateral coordination). The sensory slumper may also have poor discrimination in the touch and movement senses.

The second type of sensory-based motor differences is dyspraxia, or difficulty with *praxis* (Greek for "doing, action, practice"). Praxis is based on unconscious processing and discrimination of touch and movement sensations, as well as on conscious thought. The dyspraxic child has difficulty performing coordinated and voluntary actions.

The checklists below focus on characteristics of SPD. See the sensory-motor history questionnaire designed by Sharon A. Cermak, EdD, to help parents note patterns in their child's development, at www.out-of-sync-child.com. Also see "The Gander,"[2] a screening tool designed by Dan Shapiro, MD, with Sarah Wayland, PhD, that will help you assess and understand your child's behavior, at www.ParentChildJourney.com. After you have glanced at the next checklists, let's move on to page 25 to look at problems with self-regulation that often co-occur with inefficient sensory processing and integration.

Sensory-Based Motor Skills	Sensory Slumper (Postural Differences): "Don't want to."
Components of Movement	□ May be tense or have "loose and floppy" muscle tone, a weak grasp on objects. Has difficulty getting into and maintaining a stable position, fully flexing and extending her limbs, shifting her weight to crawl, and rotating her body to throw a ball. Slouches and sprawls.
Balance	□ Loses balance when walking or changing positions. Trips on air.
Bilateral Coordination	□ Has difficulty using both sides of the body together for jumping symmetrically, catching basket-balls, clapping, getting and staying seated. Has difficulty using one hand to assist the other, such as holding a paper while cutting, or a cup while pouring.
Unilateral Coordination	□ May not have definite hand preference. May use either hand to reach for objects or use tools such as pens and forks. May switch object from right to left hand when handling it; eat with one hand but draw with the other; manipulate scissors or tongs using both hands.
Crossing the Midline	□ Has difficulty using a hand, foot, or eye on the opposite side of the body, e.g., using just one hand to paint a horizon line across the easel, kicking a ball sideways, or reading a line across a page.

Sensory-Based Motor Skills	Sensory Fumbler (Dyspraxia): "I can't do that."
Components of Praxis	☐ May have difficulty: 1) conceiving of a new, complex action to do; 2) sequencing the steps and organizing body movements to do it; and 3) carrying out the multiple-step motor plan. May be awkward, clumsy, apparently careless (even when trying to be careful), and accident prone.
Gross-Motor Planning	☐ May have poor motor coordination and be clumsy when moving around furniture, in a crowded room, or on a busy playground or field. Has problem with stairs, obstacle courses, playground and sports equipment, and large-muscle activities such as walking, marching, crawling, and rolling. May walk on toes. Ability to learn new motor skills, such as jumping, hopping, galloping, and skipping, may develop noticeably late.
Fine-Motor Planning: Hands	☐ May have difficulty with manual tasks, including writing, buttoning, opening snack packages, using eating utensils, doing jigsaw puzzles, playing with Legos, buckling a seat belt.
Fine-Motor Planning: Eyes	☐ May have difficulty using both eyes together, tracking moving objects, focusing, and shifting gaze from far to near point. May have a problem copying from the board, keeping his place in a book, and organizing desk space. May have sloppy handwriting and poor eye-hand coordination when drawing, creating art projects, building with blocks, or tying shoes.

Sensory-Based Motor Skills	Sensory Fumbler (Dyspraxia): "I can't do that."
Fine-Motor Planning: Mouth	☐ May have difficulty sucking through a nipple or straw, chewing and swallowing, blowing bubbles, holding mouth closed. May drool excessively. May cram food into mouth and be a messy eater. May have problem articulating speech sounds and speaking clearly enough to be understood (by the age of three).

Self-Regulation Challenges

Developing self-regulation is every child's biggest job. "Very simply," says Kelly Mahler, OTD, who specializes in interoception, "self-regulation is our ability to control the way we feel and act."[3] When self-regulated, the child is generally in sync with the world. She can arouse herself to attend to what is going on around her, take appropriate action, and return to a state of equilibrium, physically, mentally, and emotionally.

Modulating (adjusting) her responses to sensations, however, may challenge the child with SPD. Thus, self-regulation may be uneven in several areas, including arousal, activity level, and attention; social and emotional functioning; and eating, toileting, and sleeping. When severe, these problems are referred to as regulatory disorders. The child may be in sync one day and out of sync the next—depending on the sensory input and her ability to adapt to it at that moment.

Note: The problems discussed below may have a sensory processing component—or they may be caused by another developmental or medical condition altogether!

AROUSAL, ACTIVITY LEVEL, AND ATTENTION

Arousal, activity level, and attention problems frequently coexist with SPD.

- Unusually high arousal and activity level: The child may become easily overwhelmed and fussy. He may be always on the go, restless, and fidgety. He may move with short and nervous gestures, play or work aimlessly, be quick-tempered and excitable, and find it impossible to stay seated. After he is hurt or upset, self-comforting may be very difficult.

- Unusually low arousal and activity level: It may be hard to "rev up." The child may move slowly and in a daze, fatigue easily, seem to lack initiative and stick-to-itiveness. She may turn away, as if disinterested in the world. She may have been an easy baby—in fact, a *too*-easy baby, who nestled into anybody's arms, rarely complained, slept more than other children, and still needed to be dressed and fed later than others.

- Inattention: The child may have a short attention span, even for activities he enjoys. He may be highly distractible and disorganized, paying attention to anticipated or unexpected sensations rather than the task at hand. Or he may quickly get overwhelmed and need a break from sensory experiences.

- Impulsivity: The child may be heedlessly energetic and impetuous. She may lack self-control in what she says and does. She may be unable to stop after starting an activity because, by the time her nervous system feels it has had enough, it has had too much. Thus, she may overeat, pour juice until it spills, run pell-mell into people, overturn toy bins, and talk out of turn.

SOCIAL AND EMOTIONAL FUNCTIONING

Other coexisting regulatory problems may be how the child feels about himself and relates to other people.

- Anxiety: By the age of three, the child may be anxious physically, emotionally, and socially. By this age, he has learned to worry, "What if Mommy squashes me into the car seat? What if I'm stuck in the back seat, where I can't see the horizon to sense where I am in space? What if she starts and stops suddenly and drives fast over speed bumps? Oh, no—what if I throw up? No car rides for me!" (Chapter 10 suggests treatments to help the child manage touch and movement sensations and to make car trips more enjoyable for everyone.)

- Poor adaptability: Attempting to control what feels overwhelming, the child may resist meeting new people or trying new activities and foods. He may have difficulty making transitions from one situation to another. He may seem stubborn and uncooperative when it is time to leave the house, come for dinner, get into or out of the tub or shower, or change from a reading to a math activity. Minor changes in routine readily upset this child who does not "go with the flow."

- Attachment problem: The child may have separation anxiety and be clingy and fearful when apart from one or two favorite caregivers. Or, as she tries to manage the sensations (smell, sound, touch) of being next to a person, she may physically avoid her parents, teachers, and others in her circle.

- Frustration: The child may struggle to accomplish tasks that peers do easily. He may give up quickly. He may find it hard to delay gratification. He may be a perfectionist and become upset when art projects, dramatic play, or homework assignments are not going as well as he expects.

- Difficulty with friendships: The child may be hard to get along with and have problems making and keeping friends. Insisting on dictating all the rules and being the winner, the best, or the first, he may be a poor game player. He may need to control his surrounding territory, be in the driver's seat, and have trouble sharing toys.

- Poor communication: As she tries to process sensations of sound, sight, and movement in a timely manner, the child may struggle verbally to articulate her speech, "get the words out," and write. She may have difficulty expressing her thoughts, feelings, and needs, not only through words but also nonverbally through gestures, body language, and facial expressions.

- Academic problems: Co-occurring with sensory challenges, the child may have difficulty learning new skills and concepts. Although bright, she may be perceived as an underachiever.

- Other emotional problems: The child may wonder why it is so hard to do what others seem to do effortlessly. He may be angry or panicky for no obvious reason. He may be inflexible, irrational, and overly sensitive to change, stress, and hurt feelings. Demanding and needy, he may seek attention in negative ways. He may be unhappy, believing and saying that he is dumb, crazy, no good, a loser, and a failure.

Lack of self-confidence and low self-esteem are telling symptoms of SPD.

EATING, TOILETING, AND SLEEPING

Because of poor self-regulation, children with SPD often have accompanying difficulties with eating, urinating/defecating (toileting), and sleeping. These are daily activities that everybody must do for oneself and that nobody else can make one do.

People do what they can to control how they experience the world. If crunchy food or a noisy toilet or a scratchy pillowcase is distressing, the child with SPD will do what is necessary to avoid it. Wouldn't you?

Eating

Preferring certain foods and protesting at others is every little child's prerogative. As she grows, the typical child learns to try and accept a variety of foods. For the child with SPD, however, settling down to eat may be a battle. Eating involves all eight sensory systems simultaneously, and one sense or more may be in revolt or out of action. (See the box "SPD's Effect on Eating," adapted from *The Out-of-Sync Child Grows Up*.)[4]

The child may be a picky eater with a limited food repertoire. Of more concern, the child may be a "problem feeder" with a severely restricted list of acceptable foods. More than two-thirds of children with SPD have feeding issues. Not only taste and smell, but also touch, proprioception, vision, and hearing affect the child's ability to eat and drink.[5] She may not have developed a sensory-based motor pattern involving sucking, swallowing, and breathing. The result is poor oral-motor skills, which affect eating solid food, trying new food, keeping food down, and digesting food, as well as relationships with family members and emotional security.

Nutritional deficits may affect her development, weight, and stamina and cause behavioral ups and downs, like a yo-yo. Usually absent from her diet, and thus from her body and brain, are essential fatty acids, B vitamins, minerals, and fat-soluble antioxidants. A child who rejects peanut butter, broccoli, beans, and sweet potatoes, for example, may get insufficient magnesium, an essential mineral. A magnesium deficiency may lead to hearing damage, auditory processing problems, muscle spasms, restless sleep, and sensory-based motor difficulties associated with frequent ear infections.

SPD's Effect on Eating

Differences in any or all eight sensory systems may cause eating problems.

* Sight: Seeing certain foods may evoke previous bad eating experiences. Or foods on the plate may touch one another, or their color may be objectionable, or they "just look gross."
* Touch: The texture, consistency, and temperature of food matter greatly. An overresponsive child may refuse to eat soft, smooth food; or lumpy, crispy, chewy, seedy, grainy food; or hot or cold food. The child with underresponsivity or poor discrimination may be uncertain about what is in his mouth and whether he has chewed sufficiently to swallow it without choking.
* Smell: Fried or aromatic food may make the overresponsive child gag or feel nauseated.
* Taste: Foods that taste very sweet, sour, bitter, spicy, or off may be disgusting. Or the child may crave sugary snacks, drink pickle juice, suck lemons, and gobble red-hot chili.
* Sound: Hearing others take bites, chew, slurp, and swallow may be painful. This condition is known as misophonia, literally, "hatred of sounds." (See page 61.)

* Body position: Positioning his hands to use utensils, getting food to his mouth, and chewing may be difficult because of inefficient processing of sensations coming from muscles and joints.
* Movement: Staying seated may challenge the child if he has low postural tone, or if he cannot sense whether he is sitting up or falling off his chair. Or he may crave movement and be unable to sit quietly for long.
* Internal organs: Eating or even the anticipation of eating may be distressing. An overresponsive child may dread the feeling of a full stomach, for example, or avoid foods that may cause an upset stomach or diarrhea.

A deficiency in zinc (found in eggs, peanuts, bran, cocoa, etc.) may affect the "out-of-zinc" child's sense of smell and taste and, thus, her interest in food. It may also lead to low muscle tone, auditory and visual problems, rashes, and fly-away hair.

Here are suggestions to improve your child's eating, from nutritionist Kelly Dorfman, author of *Cure Your Child with Food*:

* Eliminate junk food, which offer empty calories.
* Eliminate juice and replace with water.
* Eliminate irritants, which may include chocolate, citrus, carbonated soda, dairy products, and food coloring.
* Add nutritional supplements, especially omega-3 fats, found in flaxseeds, walnuts, and salmon. (The brain is made up of about 60 percent fat and needs the right kind of fat to function well.)
* Offer a vibrating toothbrush or facial/oral massager to desensitize lips and mouth and to provide deep pressure that increases tolerance of other sensory input.
* Consider occupational therapy with a sensory integration approach (OT-SI).

• Support your child's daily functioning with what
Lindsey Biel, coauthor of *Raising a Sensory Smart Child*,
calls a "sensory-enriched life" (see chapter 11).

Toileting

Just as nobody can make a child eat, nobody can make a
child poop. The sensations involved in this job may overwhelm a
child with SPD. (See the box "SPD's Effect on Toilet Training.")

Part of the pooping problem is with the food that the child
takes in. What goes in must come out. Sometimes what goes
in gets stuck on the way out; sometimes it gushes out. The
picky eater who has a limited diet and declines healthful foods
with naturally bright color, varied texture, and lots of fiber—
the stuff of stool, if you will—is likely to have chronic constipa-
tion or diarrhea.

SPD's Effect on Toilet Training

Differences in the child's response to sensations may cause toileting
problems.

* Sight: Seeing stool may make the child squeamish, or she may
  want to examine it right away and for a long time, since she
  "made it."
* Touch: The overresponsive child may avoid pooping because it is
  wet and sticky. The underresponsive child who is unaware of wetness may not develop efficient bladder control. (Thick disposable
  diapers that carry wetness away to keep the child comfortably dry
  are part of the problem!) The sensory craver may actually like how
  poop feels in pants . . . or hands.
* Smell: Some children will be repelled by the smell and resist going
  near a toilet. Others may be interested in the odor because it
  came from their own body.

* Sound: A noisy flushing toilet may overwhelm the child with sensitive hearing. Another child may repeatedly flush because he likes hearing (and seeing) the action in the toilet.
* Body position: An inefficient sense of body parts and muscles may make it hard for the child to "hold it." A postural challenge may be in staying poised on the toilet seat.
* Movement: The child who is sedentary because of difficulty moving his body may also have difficulty moving his bowels. The child may feel unbalanced and ungrounded, as if he is falling off the toilet—or, worse, in.
* Internal organs: The child may not recognize bladder or bowel fullness. Or the child may feel he has to use the toilet far more often than other children do.

The child may develop problems with bladder control as well. He may wait too long to use the toilet, frequently wet his clothes, and become a chronic bed wetter.

Suggestions from Maria Wheeler, a behavior specialist and author of *Toilet Training for Individuals with Autism and Other Developmental Issues*, include:

* Plenty of water, fiber, and active movement throughout the day.
* A visual toileting schedule.
* Comfortable clothing during toilet training.
* A step stool under the child's feet to help him feel grounded while on the toilet.
* Working with an OT, nutritionist, or other professional with expertise in bladder and bowel problems.

Sleeping

Eating problems, toileting problems . . . and then, at the end of a long day, problems with falling asleep, staying asleep, and awakening may beset the child and family. Weary parents may wonder if SPD ever rests. (See the box "SPD's Effect on Sleeping," adapted from *The Out-of-Sync Child Grows Up*.)[6]

The child may need long naps or may never nap even if exhausted. As a sleep problem is often caused by a separation problem, she may want to sleep with her parents. She may be unable to comfort herself to sleep or may constantly awaken during the night.

Coming full circle, disturbed sleep leads to inefficient sensory feedback and ineffective self-regulation. It increases arousal as the child's body tries to fight sleepiness, including higher levels of stress, anxiety, depression, irritability, and anger. It decreases attention, memory, judgment, and problem-solving while performing daily tasks and doing schoolwork.

Sensory integration treatment addresses poor self-regulation, the underlying problem. Meanwhile, thinking about the sensory experiences that help or hamper a good night's sleep can give parents more strategies. Problem-solving the sensory need and adding sensory solutions can help the whole family sleep better.

SPD's Effect on Sleeping

Certain sensations may disturb the child's sleep.

* Touch: Pajamas and bed linens may feel scratchy. Blankets may make the child uncomfortably hot or not warm enough. The mattress may feel lumpy (think of "The Princess and the Pea"). Blankets may feel too heavy or not heavy enough.
* Sound: Sounds preventing sleep include someone's breathing or snoring; house creaks, air-conditioning and heating motors; or rain, crickets, and traffic outside.
* Sight: Streetlights, lamplight, or light-emitting diodes (LEDs) of electronic devices in standby mode may keep the child awake.

* Movement: Passive, unexpected activity may bother the sleeper, as when a bedmate turns over and the mattress shifts.
* Body and muscles: The child's active movement quota for the day has not been met, so the body is not ready for sleep.
* Smell: The pillowcase may smell wrong, especially after its familiar, ripe scent has been washed out.
* Internal organs: Poor appetite, irregular bowel movements, stomach "butterflies," uneven heart rate, etc., may make it hard to fall and stay asleep (and vice versa!).

Until this problem is "put to rest," try these ideas to help a child sleep:

* During the day—plenty of active movement, such as jogging and carrying laundry baskets; dietary supplements that calm the brain, such as magnesium, essential fatty acids, and GABA (gamma-aminobutyric acid); no foods with additives, including aspartame, MSG, and artificial colors, which excite the brain.
* Before going to bed—a warm bath or shower and then right into bed; no TV or electronic devices for a couple of hours before bedtime.
* In bed—one great story; a back massage and deep joint compression to the shoulders, arms, and legs; a tight tuck-in under a weighted blanket; and saying, "Just *pretend* to sleep."
* After the tuck-in—a night-light if the child fears the dark; peaceful music, e.g., Bach or Mozart adagios; white noise such as the sound of rain or waves; and your own parental resolve!

SPD is a primary concern because it affects not only the child but also the whole family. Adults can make children feel more secure and able to explore "just right" sensory experiences by acknowledging bothersome sensations and saying, "Lots of folks think dog spit is disgusting. Let's find a sink to rinse it off." Or, "Some people don't think flushing a toilet is loud, and others think it sounds like being under Niagara Falls, and I can help."

Additionally, a sensory-enriched life, nutritional supplements, and OT are some of the treatments that may help (see chapter 11). OT reduces maladaptive behaviors and helps a child get in sync so he can develop more mature coping strategies and socially appropriate behaviors.

Please note: *While many children with SPD have behavior problems, most children with behavior problems do not have SPD!* Careful diagnosis is imperative to determine which symptoms are related to sensory processing problems and which are not, for every child is occasionally out of sync.

Who Has SPD?

Some people have a poorly integrated neurological system, some have an excellent one, and the rest of us fall somewhere in the middle.

Think about people who are graceful and popular, such as athletes, charismatic politicians, and "easy" children. These people may be blessed with exceptionally efficient sensory processing.

Now, think about people you know who have problems functioning in certain aspects of their lives. They may be clumsy, have few friends, or seem to lack common sense. They may have SPD.

SPD is on a continuum. The child with mild SPD is slightly impaired. The way he processes sensory information is a "difference," not a disorder. For example, he may prefer blander food and quieter activities or spicier food and more roughhousing than other children do. He may find ways to compensate—and his sensory processing problem is frequently overlooked. He will probably function better at home and in school with support from his family, teachers, and perhaps other professionals.

The child with moderate SPD shows more symptoms. He may need substantial support.

The child with severe SPD shows many symptoms. Succeeding in ordinary childhood occupations—waking up, eating, dressing, playing, going to school, having a conversation, bathing, falling asleep—may be greatly impaired. His out-of-sync sensory processing is not merely a "difference"; it has become a disorder, and the child may require very substantial support.

Rondalyn V. Whitney, PhD, explains that sensory processing differences can be part of a cluster of symptoms that may result in difficulty with reading, or kicking a ball, or tying shoelaces.[7] If several differences are present, they can mount up to meeting the list of criteria for a more involved disorder. Think of the flu: if you have a sore throat but nothing else, it is not the flu. Add chills, fever, aching muscles, and other symptoms, and as they add up, they meet the more significant diagnosis of the flu. Teasing apart the symptoms helps parents and professionals clarify the best treatment.

We know that SPD intensifies the bigger problems of children with the disorders, syndromes, and environmental conditions mentioned in chapter 3. We know that some children with neurological "soft signs," who are not regarded as having diagnosable problems, also have SPD. For all these children, remediation through occupational therapy has an overall positive effect.

What percentage of children is challenged by inefficient sensory processing? Statistics are slippery and depend on the criteria used. Prevalence studies vary from 5 percent[8] to 16.5 percent.[9]

Occupational therapists commonly note that approximately 80 percent of their clients are boys. Girls are just as likely as boys to have neurological problems, including sensory, attentional, and learning disabilities. Girls, however, often do not display the same behavior problems that attract attention, so they tend to go unnoticed—and to fall through the cracks.

Should we be alarmed by the increasing numbers of children identified as having SPD? Are we indiscriminately sticking labels on children? Are we "just looking for something wrong"?

No, no, no!

In fact, identifying children with SPD is a positive step. As we learn more about the mechanics of the human brain, we are finally understanding why some children are out of sync. And now we can do something to help!

Hope Is at Hand

Having looked at this chapter, you should be getting a feel for how SPD can get in a child's way. If you (and the teacher, spouse, mother-in-law, et al.) checked the same boxes, you may believe you have an out-of-sync child. You may be asking: Is my child's development out of my hands? Will my child become an out-of-sync adult?

Not necessarily. Your child may develop into a self-regulating, functioning grown-up if he or she receives understanding, support, and intervention.

Designed to correct or prevent the child's developmental delays or disabilities, intervention usually comes in the form of occupational therapy in a sensory integration framework, OT-SI. (See chapter 10.) For the child with severe SPD, treatment is crucial. For the child with moderate or mild SPD, treatment can effect wonderful changes.

Treatment helps the child now to build a strong foundation for the future, when life becomes more demanding and complex. Without treatment, SPD persists as a lifelong problem. Indeed, *the child will not grow out of SPD but will grow into it.*

Young children respond well to OT-SI because their nervous systems are still flexible, or "plastic" (from the Greek *plastikos*, meaning moldable). Plasticity means that brain functioning is not fixed; it can change or be changed. As children grow, their brains become less malleable and unusual reactions to sensations become more established. However, if your child is an adolescent, do not give up hope! Older children and adults do benefit from therapy, too. It is never too late.

Treatment helps the child integrate and process all the senses so that they work together. When the child *actively* engages in meaningful activities that provide the intensity, duration, and quality of sensation his central nervous system (CNS) needs, his adaptive behavior improves. Adaptive behavior, in turn, leads to better sensory processing. The child becomes able to plan, organize, and carry out what he needs and wants to do. Without treatment, severe SPD may hamper his life in countless ways.

Treatment helps the child develop skills to engage successfully in social situations. Without it, SPD interferes with the child's friendships and all-important play.

Treatment gives the child the tools to become a more efficient learner. Without it, SPD interferes with perceptual skills and the ability to learn, at home, in school, and abroad.

Treatment improves emotional well-being and self-confidence. Without it, the child who believes she is incompetent may develop into an adult with low self-esteem.

Treatment improves family relationships. As the child responds to sensory challenges with growing self-control, home life becomes more pleasant. Parents learn to provide consistent discipline and to enjoy their child. Relatives become more empathetic and less critical, and siblings resent the out-of-sync child less. Without treatment, SPD can interfere with the interactions and coping skills of everyone in the family.

Johnny is an example of a child who greatly benefited from early intervention. When he was a preschooler, SPD affected his ability to move, play, learn, and relate to others. It affected his posture and balance, hearing and vision, food preferences and sleep patterns. He was fearful, angry, inflexible, and lonely.

Johnny's feet never left the ground because movement made him uncomfortable. He would watch but not join his schoolmates in playground activities. He always carried a stick, as a buffer against the world. When someone approached, he would brandish the stick and holler, "You're fired!" His sole pleasure was curling up in the quiet corner, peering at a book.

Johnny was one of the first children we screened for SPD at St. Columba's Nursery School. We shared our findings with his parents and suggested OT, mentioning that early intervention could prevent later problems.

Listening to us, his father folded his arms, scowled, and shook his head. His mother wept and said, "This is all a bad dream."

Although skeptical, his parents decided to take our advice. They took Johnny to a pediatric occupational therapist twice a week. Working with the therapist and his teachers, they devised a sensory-enriched life with activities at home and in school to help him become as competent as he could be.

Gradually, Johnny began to participate in some activities. He did not learn to relish messy play or a rowdy game of tag, but he did learn to paint at the easel and jump down from a step. He stopped carrying his stick in self-defense. He started to use his "indoor" voice instead of bellowing. He found a friend, and then two. He was becoming a real kid.

By the age of ten, Johnny turned into a dream come true. He played soccer and basketball. As a Boy Scout, he enjoyed camping and climbing rocks. He read a book every week, for pleasure. Everyone wanted to be his friend, because he was reliable and sensitive—in all the right ways. His teacher said, "I wish I had twenty-four other Johnnys in my classroom."

Decades later, Johnny is a journalist living and traveling in Europe with his girlfriend. His SPD, once severe, is now mild. He still eats carefully, feels uncomfortable in crowds, avoids escalators, and tends to be a perfectionist. But nobody's perfect!

Not every out-of-sync child will have Johnny's success. Most children do improve, however, when their parents take action. Here are some suggestions:

- Get information and share it with pediatricians, teachers, and other caregivers, when appropriate.
- Although difficult to do, accept that the child does not fit your mental image of the perfect child; acknowledge that it is okay and sometimes preferable to have differing abilities.
- Provide the child with a sensory-enriched life (see chapter 11).
- Be patient, consistent, and supportive.
- Help the child take control of his or her body and life.
- Read *The Out-of-Sync Child Grows Up* to learn what happens next.

The journey may be long. It may be expensive. It will certainly be frustrating at times. But the journey will also be wonderful and exciting as you learn to help your son or daughter succeed in the occupation of childhood.

Hope is at hand.

3

Does Your Child Have
Another Diagnosis?

This chapter considers other diagnoses that frequently co-occur with SPD. Reading about these "look-alikes" and "overlappers" may especially interest you if you know or suspect that SPD is not your child's sole difference. Then chapter 4 will explain typical sensory processing and integration and what can go amiss.

A democratic problem, SPD affects people of all ages, races, and cognitive skills, all over the world. Diverse populations include those with autism spectrum disorders, those with cerebral palsy, premature babies, sensory-deprived children in overseas orphanages, and highly gifted people. While these individuals may not seem to have much in common, they frequently experience similar problems in processing sensations.

SPD does not cause—but certainly does complicate—other conditions. The more difficulty a child has in interpreting and using sensory input, the more problematic behavioral output will be, such as moving, eating, relating to others, expressing one's thoughts, or keeping calm when lightly touched.

What SPD Is Not: "Look-Alike" Symptoms (LD, ADHD, and ASD)

Determining that a child has SPD can bewilder parents as well as professionals. While SPD can stand alone, it often coexists with many other developmental disabilities. And SPD can look like—and be mistaken for—many other conditions, because many sensory symptoms are common to them all.

So how can one tell the difference between SPD and other disabilities? *The red flags are a child's unusual responses to touching and being touched, or to moving and being moved.*

For example, if a child refuses hugs, cannot jump, is a picky eater, or struggles to write, he may have SPD. If he has difficulty staying focused not only on tasks he dislikes but also on activities he enjoys, he may have SPD. If he constantly fidgets and squirms, he may have SPD. If he has few friends, he may have SPD.

But—might something else be going on? Yes, indeed! Additional diagnoses may be different problems: attention deficit hyperactivity disorder (ADHD), autism spectrum disorder (ASD), and/or learning disabilities (LD). Prevalence studies show:

- About one in 16 children (6.25 percent) has SPD.[1]
- About one in 9 children (9.4 percent) has ADHD[2] and about 40 percent of them also have SPD.[3]
- About one in 54 children (1.85 percent) has autism,[4] and about 95 percent of them also have SPD.[5]
- Between one in 20 (5 percent) and one in 11 children (9 percent) has LD.[6] For the purposes of this book, let's say that the prevalence is one in 15 (6.66 percent) and that many of them also have SPD.

The overlapping circles in the diagram illustrate—in a decidedly unscientific way—the general relationship of these four common problems.

The descriptions below provide information about these look-alike conditions that the child may have *instead of SPD or alongside SPD*. Several other conditions with which SPD may coexist are then briefly described.

HOW FOUR COMMON PROBLEMS MAY OVERLAP

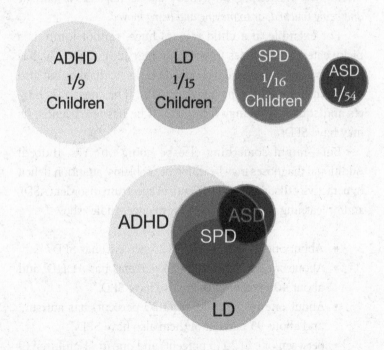

LEARNING DISABILITY (LD)

One look-alike is a learning disability (LD). This can be defined in many ways.

1) Simple definition: A learning disability is difficulty in reading, writing, mathematics, and coordinating movements, despite one's intelligence and motivation.

2) Clinical definition: A learning disability is a problem in processing information that causes difficulties mastering academic skills and strategies. A breakdown occurs in one of the four steps involved in learning: input (taking in information from the senses), integration (processing and interpreting the information), memory (using, storing, and retrieving the information), and output (sending out the information through language or motor activities).

3) Formal definition: In the United States, our federal law, *Individuals with Disabilities Education Improvement Act of 2004 (IDEA 04),*[7] defines a specific learning disability as "a disorder in one or more of the basic psychological processes involved in understanding or in using language, spoken or written, that may manifest itself in an imperfect ability to listen, think, speak, read, write, spell, or to do mathematical calculations."

According to this formal definition, SPD is not a learning disability. However, SPD can certainly lead to future learning disabilities when it affects the child's auditory, visual, and motor skills and his ability to process and sequence information. In turn, LD can exacerbate sensory processing challenges. At the moment, having only SPD does not qualify a child for free, appropriate services at school, such as occupational, speech-language, and physical therapy. But a student with SPD can receive services when his family and teachers demonstrate that his sensory differences coexist with other qualifying problems that limit his ability to learn. The most common qualifying problems are those with the "three Rs"—reading (dyslexia and hyperlexia), 'riting (dysgraphia), and 'rithmetic (dyscalculia).

Dyslexia ("difficulty" plus "words") is the problem in the way different brain parts simultaneously process sight, sound, and movement—the sensory components of reading. The timing is out of sync, preventing instantaneous, automatic word recognition.

Hyperlexia ("over" plus "words") is unusually advanced reading ability and an intense fascination with letters and numbers at a very young age, without reading comprehension and verbal communication skills. It may be a sign that a child is gifted or has autism—or both. Children may have strong auditory and visual memory but be overresponsive to ordinary sounds and sights and have other differences as well.

Dysgraphia ("difficulty" plus "writing") is a disability in transcription, which involves handwriting, typing, and spelling. Sensations of touch, sight, and movement are not integrated, resulting in poor fine-motor coordination. Dysgraphia is seen in 40 percent of children with SPD and shares common brain abnormalities with children who have autism and ADHD.[8] The child may awkwardly grip the pencil and write illegibly. She may mumble while writing, omit words, make grammatical errors, and have problems organizing and expressing thoughts on the page, even when those thoughts are brilliant.

Dyscalculia ("difficulty" plus "counting") causes problems with numbers, time, and space. Sensations of sight, sound, movement, and body awareness are involved with math concepts (subtracting, counting money); visual-spatial concepts (reading graphs, judging distances); auditory skills (recalling dates, playing music); time (reading analog clocks, being punctual); speed (running, biking); and body awareness (assessing the length of one's stride or reach; knowing left from right).

What can you do to help children with dyslexia, hyperlexia, dysgraphia, and dyscalculia?

- Consider OT to incorporate multisensory treatment that integrates sight, sound, touch, and movement experiences.
- Consider a developmental vision evaluation by a developmental optometrist. To find one, go to the College of Optometrists in Vision Development at www.COVD.org.
- At home and school, get kids moving! Reading, writing, and arithmetic involve the whole body, not merely the eyes and hands. Have children count their jumps, climb ladder rungs, hit a tetherball, and shoot baskets. Read stories and poetry aloud. Count coins. Stir cookie dough. Physical activities to develop and enhance sensory and perceptual skills will make a positive difference. (See chapters 11 and 12. Also see my book *Growing an In-Sync Child*.)
- Visit www.ldaamerica.org, the website of the Learning Disabilities Association, to find detailed information and treatment recommendations.

ATTENTION DEFICIT HYPERACTIVITY DISORDER (ADHD)

SPD is not the same as its look-alike ADHD. Sometimes behaviors look similar, but the underlying reasons vary. Research is illuminating how sensory differences happen all over the brain and how the brains of people with neurological problems vary. (For more about the brain, see appendix A.)

Different as they are, the two problems may simultaneously

affect the out-of-sync child (or adult). About 40 percent of children with SPD have ADHD, and vice versa.[9] According to the *DSM-5*, ADHD's symptoms are inattention, or hyperactivity and impulsivity, or a combination of them all. Six symptoms of inattention and/or of hyperactivity and impulsivity must be present to make a diagnosis of ADHD.

These symptoms are also seen in children with SPD, so let's ask, "Is it ADHD—or SPD?" When a child feels restless and wants the world to move faster . . . does he have ADHD or could he be a sensory craver? When she is easily distracted by stimuli around her . . . is it ADHD or could she be a sensory avoider? When he cannot sit still . . . is it ADHD or could he be a sensory slumper or fumbler? When she seems not to listen . . . is it ADHD or does she discriminate sounds differently from most people?

Furthermore, these symptoms are not exclusive to ADHD or to SPD. All sorts of children are easily distracted, lose things, and cannot sit still. Patricia S. Lemer, a wise educational diagnostician, has designed a chart showing that the very same symptoms show up in the behavior of children with ADHD, *and* with SPD, *and* with learning-related visual problems, *and* with allergies and nutritional deficits, *and*—no surprise—with the "condition" of being a typical child under the age of seven!

Alternative Diagnoses to ADHD

Patricia S. Lemer

Symptoms	ADHD	SPD	Visual Problems	Nutrition / Allergies	Typical Child Under 7
Inattention (at least 6 necessary). The child OFTEN:					
Fails to give close attention to details or makes careless mistakes	✔	✔	✔	✔	
Has difficulty sustaining attention in tasks or play activities	✔	✔	✔	✔	✔
Does not listen when spoken to directly	✔	✔	✔	✔	
Does not follow through on instructions or fails to finish work	✔	✔	✔	✔	✔
Has difficulty organizing activities, sequencing tasks, and managing time	✔	✔	✔	✔	✔
Avoids, dislikes, or is reluctant to engage in tasks requiring sustained mental effort	✔	✔	✔	✔	✔

Symptoms	ADHD	SPD	Visual Problems	Nutrition / Allergies	Typical Child Under 7
Loses things	✔	✔	✔	✔	✔
Is distracted by extraneous stimuli	✔	✔	✔	✔	✔
Is forgetful in daily activities	✔	✔	✔	✔	
Hyperactivity and Impulsivity (at least 6 necessary). The child OFTEN:					
Fidgets with hands or feet, or squirms in seat	✔	✔	✔	✔	✔
Has difficulty remaining seated when required to do so	✔	✔	✔	✔	✔
Runs or climbs excessively	✔	✔		✔	✔
Has difficulty playing quietly	✔	✔		✔	
Is "on the go"; is uncomfortable being still	✔	✔		✔	✔
Talks excessively	✔	✔	✔	✔	
Blurts out answers to questions before they have been completed	✔	✔	✔	✔	

Symptoms	ADHD	SPD	Visual Problems	Nutrition / Allergies	Typical Child Under 7
Has difficulty awaiting turn	✔	✔	✔	✔	✔
Interrupts or intrudes on others			✔	✔	✔

Discerning the differences between ADHD and SPD (and other conditions) matters. Lucy Jane Miller, PhD, one of the world's principal investigators in the field of sensory processing, has collaborated with other OTs to define the underlying neurological and physiological foundations of SPD. Their goals have included: 1) distinguishing SPD from ADHD and other disabilities, and 2) determining the best treatment for children with different types of SPD.

Their research has found that many children with only SPD differ from children with only ADHD in their responses to unexpected sensations, such as light touches, loud noises, flickering lights, strong smells, and being tilted backward in a chair.[10] Children with ADHD tend to alert to these novel sensations and then, like most people, habituate—i.e., become easily accustomed—to them. Life goes on.

Some children with SPD, however, may not alert to these everyday sensations. Life does not appear to affect sensory stragglers much.

Other children with SPD may respond differently, being continually on alert and not becoming accustomed to the sensations. Life affects sensory avoiders too much.

Outside the research laboratory, parents and teachers may notice other differences between SPD and ADHD. Mim Ochsenbein, pediatric OT and director of education at STAR

Institute, points out some of these dissimilarities. For instance, many children with SPD prefer the "same old, same old" in a familiar and predictable environment, while children with ADHD prefer novelty and diversion. Many children with SPD have adequate impulse control and can calm down and focus when they get the "just-right" sensory input. Meanwhile, children with ADHD often have poor impulse control regardless of sensory input; what helps them calm down and focus is constant novelty.

Determining the child's specific differences is important in order to choose the best treatment. Treatment for ADHD may be:

- Cognitive behavior therapy (helping a person learn to think before doing).
- Medications that improve attention and impulsivity by helping normal brain chemicals work better. Some medications may also help children with SPD.
- Parent training for families with SPD and ADHD, helping mothers and fathers raise their children with nonpunitive, caring, and realistic expectations.
- Occupational therapy focusing on sensory integration and a sensory-enriched life with purposeful activities that help both types of children while addressing different problems.

To learn more, visit Children and Adults with ADHD (CHADD) at www.chadd.org and get support at www .ADDitudemag.com.

AUTISM (AUTISM SPECTRUM DISORDERS—ASD)

Autism, a third look-alike, is a complex, multisystem disorder affecting the body and the brain. According to the *DSM-5*, autism has qualitative impairments in three areas. (The term "qualitative" refers to understanding behavior in natural settings, such as home and school, through observations and verbal descriptions. In contrast, "quantitative" refers to findings based on numerical facts.) These three areas are:

- Social interaction, with impaired use of nonverbal behaviors, such as pointing or waving; limited relationships; and lack of social/emotional reciprocity, such as feeling sad when someone else is sad, or laughing at jokes.
- Communication, with delayed speaking, difficulty with conversations, and limited make-believe play.
- Hyper- or hypo-reactivity to sensory input or unusual interest in sensory aspects of the environment.

Not only sensory modulation challenges with over- and underresponsivity (called "hyper- or hypo-reactivity" in the *DSM-5*), but also sensory discrimination and sensory-based motor skills (for some reason, not included in the *DSM-5*) are usually huge problems for people with autism. Problems with sensations are sometimes overlooked or downplayed and may be their biggest challenges.

According to the *DSM-5*, some children with ASD have an intellectual disability (ID), and others are intellectually at or above average. Some are mildly impaired and may need a little support to navigate the social world, to communicate, or to develop more adaptive behaviors with the sensory world (Level 1). Some are moderately impaired and need substantial support (Level 2). Some are severely impaired and need *very* substantial support (Level 3).

See the box to read how twin brothers with autism receive

support at home as their grandparents, Abuela and Abuelo, provide "just-right" sensory strategies. Cezar has Level 1 autism, no intellectual disability, and the need for some support. Felipe has Level 3 autism, an intellectual disability, and the need for very substantial support.

How Sensory-Rich Strategies Help Two Boys with ASD

Cezar: ASD, Level 1, without ID	Felipe: ASD, Level 3, with ID
Cezar, ten, and his twin brother, Felipe, come home from school. Cezar has mild SD. He shrugs off his backpack, hangs it carefully on a hook, hugs Abuelo, and heads for the kitchen. Abuela notices that Cezar looks sad and that he has been chewing his T-shirt collar as usual. She gives him a long hug and rocks him from side to side. The deep pressure and lateral movement are soothing, and he relaxes in her arms. She says, "I made churros. They taste better than T-shirts." Cezar straddles a therapy ball and bounces up and down while crunching on a churro. Eventually, he says, "In math class, teacher got mad. I was not listening." Abuela asks, "What were you thinking about?" "Batteries," he says. Abuela offers him another churro. "Tell me about batteries." He explains his emerging idea to use solar power for recharging batteries. She listens and nods. He feels reassured and loved. He looks at her smiling face and says, "I wish you were my teacher."	Felipe, ten, has severe ASD and an intellectual disability. Abuelo greets his grandsons at the door. He gives Cezar a hug and helps Felipe disentangle himself from his backpack. Abuelo hangs it on a hook and leads the boy swiftly to the toilet. (Felipe avoids the school washroom because it is noisy, smelly, and not like home.) When he is done, Felipe vocalizes a sound like "Abba!" and Abuelo goes in to coach him. Abuelo points to pictures on a wall chart and says, "Flush. Zip. Wash hands." Then they go to the kitchen. Abuela gives Felipe a big hug, helps him position himself on his therapy ball, and offers him a gluten-free plain pretzel. (Felipe does not like churros because their ridges confuse his tongue.) While Felipe gnaws on the pretzel, Abuelo stands behind him to keep him on the ball and presses down, down, on his shoulders to get him bouncing. Felipe grins and shouts happy sounds. His family helps him feel in sync.

What is the cause of autism? Everyone wants to know. The disorder seems to be caused by a combination of various genes (not all identified yet) and stressors coming from the environment, such as medications, pregnancy complications, electromagnetic fields, and toxins in our water, air, and food.

Patricia Lemer, author of *Outsmarting Autism*, points to scientists' mounting interest in the influence of the gut microbiome. The gut microbiome is all the microorganisms, bacteria, viruses, protozoa, and fungi that live in one's gastrointestinal tract.[11] Usually, when the gut is in tune, so is the brain.

Ms. Lemer notes that typically the "brain combines incoming sensory information simultaneously, just as a conductor enables individual instruments of an orchestra to make one beautiful sound. The 'beautiful sounds' of efficient sensory processing are focused attention, enjoyable learning, and appropriate behavior."[12] The gut and brain of children with ASD and SPD, however, may be out of tune. (To learn how harmony between the gut and the nervous system, via the vagal nerve, is essential to keep us "humming" and feeling safe, read about the polyvagal theory of Stephen Porges, PhD, at www.stephen porges.com.)[13]

Just as the causes of autism are being rigorously researched, so are its effects. Research illuminates why atypical structure and function of the brains of people with autism result in atypical behaviors. For example, a frequent research finding is a small corpus callosum (the connection between the right and left sides of the brain) in some children with autism, affecting the children's auditory system and language development.[14]

Using functional and structural brain imaging, researchers are now able to "see" the brain's connections and activity. Astonishing images illustrate sensory processing as it is happening inside the heads of children with and without autism. For instance, Elysa Marco, MD, and colleagues at the University of California/San Francisco and Cortica Healthcare have found that children with SPD have clear and measurable structural differences in their brain connectivity.[15]

Follow-up studies show that children with ASD and SPD look similar in some ways and different in others. What the children's brains have in common is irregularity in processing and connecting sensations. The underconnectivity theory explains this irregular communication between the front and back parts of the brain, which interferes with synchronized brain activity and, thus, with behavior.

Each child with autism has a unique pattern of sensory differences. One child may have excellent visual discrimination and be a talented artist but have poor auditory discrimination and little language. Another child may have superb auditory skills and enjoy songs and stories but have poor visual discrimination and meager motor skills.

For some, the capacity to regulate touch, movement, sound, and visual stimuli will always be troublesome. A well-known spokesperson for autism, Temple Grandin, PhD, describes the torment of sensory stimulation. As a child, being touched made her feel like a wild animal until she designed a squeeze machine—her "hug box"—to satisfy her normal craving to be held. Ordinary sounds still make her heart race and ears hurt, unless she "shuts off" her ears by engaging in rhythmic, stereotypical autistic behavior. Whereas little Temple avoided touch and sound sensations, she craved visual sensations. "I loved striped shirts and Day-Glo paint," she writes, "and I loved to watch supermarket sliding doors go back and forth."[16] Equipped with intense visualization skills and simpatico with animals, Dr. Grandin grew up to earn her doctorate in animal science.

Today she specializes in the design of humane livestock-handling facilities.

Environmental sensitivity can be a bonus and lead to remarkably satisfying professional lives. Among civilization's most creative computer wizards, composers, inventors, painters, writers, actors, mathematicians, engineers, scientists, doctors, teachers, and therapists are people who have used their "extrasensory" abilities to benefit the world. And where in the world would we be without them?

Understanding how sensory and motor problems complicate the child's daily life is crucial for designing an appropriate intervention program. Parents must ensure that their child's treatment includes strategies for coping with overwhelming sensations and individualized sensory-motor activities. (See chapter 11.)

To learn more about ASD, visit the Autism Society of America at autism-society.org.

Other Conditions Involving SPD

In addition to autism, attentional problems, and learning disabilities, numerous other conditions involve sensory processing challenges. (Chapter 8 is about vision; chapter 9 is about hearing and speech/language.) Various mental health problems, genetic syndromes, allergies, and several other "overlappers" are briefly discussed below.

MENTAL HEALTH DIAGNOSES

Many mental health problems can emerge in childhood. SPD may cause, overlap with, and contribute to psychological and emotional issues. Research suggests that sensory and motor

challenges are often present before the full-blown expression
of childhood disorders, indicating a vulnerable brain state.[17]
Furthermore, sensory and motor impairments in childhood are
associated with anxiety and other emotional difficulties in
adulthood.[18]

If the sensory and motor difficulties are neither recognized
nor addressed early with sensory-based intervention, underlying vulnerabilities in the brain may exacerbate conditions
such as:

- Anxiety disorder
- Bipolar disorder
- Depression
- Obsessive-compulsive disorder
- Schizophrenia
- Selective mutism

Sadly, SPD is often misinterpreted as a psychological problem. Distinguishing SPD from mental and emotional disorders
is as important as distinguishing it from ADHD and LD, because the treatments vary greatly. Psychotherapy, or "talk therapy," along with medication and occupational therapy to
address everyday functioning, may help all children showing
sensory symptoms. However, psychotherapy alone will not resolve the actual sensory problems.

GENETIC SYNDROMES

It is estimated that as many as 18 percent of children with
SPD have a genetic contributor from a neurodevelopment-
related gene.[19] In addition, many known genetic conditions can

have sensory differences as a clinical feature. Here are a few examples.

Down syndrome is a congenital disorder caused by an extra chromosome, causing altered development of the brain and body, cognitive impairment, and sensory problems. Common problems include poor muscle tone and challenges with fine-motor and gross-motor skills that affect movement and coordination, play and self-care, speech and eating.

Fragile X syndrome, the first known genetic cause of autism, is the result of a mutation in a gene on the X chromosome. Children with fragile X, almost always boys, have sensory over-responsivity and sensory-based motor difficulties.

Less common congenital syndromes coexisting with SPD, which may be overlooked or misdiagnosed, include:

- Angelman
- CHARGE
- Dandy-Walker
- Ehlers-Danlos
- Prader-Willi
- Rett
- Russell-Silver
- Smith-Lemli-Opitz
- Williams
- X and Y chromosomal variations

Some characteristics are avoiding or craving sensory input, particularly sight, sound, touch, and movement; decreased sensitivity to pain; sleeping and eating problems; low muscle tone; motor coordination problems with crawling, balancing, walking, and talking; and problems with sustaining attention and regulating arousal level. Occupational therapy can improve motor, social, and language skills. Other therapies, including physical therapy and speech/language therapy, may also help, especially when taking a sensory integration approach.

ALLERGIES

SPD often coexists with allergies. The child may suffer from allergic reactions to dust, pollens, molds, grass, pet dander, and, of course, foods. The casein in dairy products and the gluten in wheat, while not "true" allergens like potentially life-threatening peanuts or shellfish, can cause sensitivities. These sensitivities may lead to chronic health problems with digestion, eczema, asthma, and other issues. Additionally, the chemicals in food, medicines, and the air we inhale may be toxic for the child with a sensitive system. These allergens can harm his developing nervous system, exacerbating sensory processing challenges and causing learning and behavior problems.

In her classic book, *Is This Your Child?*, Doris Rapp, MD, discusses the predominant symptoms of allergies, including the allergic nose rub ("allergic salute"), red circles under the eyes ("allergic shiners"), irritability, depression, and aggression, and under- or overresponsivity to sensory stimulation, particularly sound and touch.

Medicine is not usually the antidote. The solution for many children is identifying and eliminating irritating foods, such as milk or wheat, and environmental irritants, such as stuffed animals and mold. Try it—and watch how many symptoms associated with allergies and sensory processing disorders clear up dramatically and without side effects.

More Look-Alikes and Overlappers

In varying degrees, sensory processing problems overlap with every physical and psychological condition, even the common cold. When your senses of smell, taste, movement, etc., are temporarily under siege, you suffer—and certainly appreciate good health when the cold is over and your senses get back in sync.

Of course, not all ailments are so insignificant and brief as a cold. Here are a few more lasting conditions that may look like or overlap with SPD.

- Fetal alcohol spectrum disorder is a preventable, non-genetic disability affecting the baby whose mother drinks alcohol during pregnancy. Symptoms include low body weight, poor coordination, and vision and hearing problems. This is often a "hidden" problem in children adopted from foreign countries where alcohol use is poorly regulated.
- Misophonia ("hatred of sounds") is a hearing condition in which repetitive human sounds such as breathing, chewing, and slurping cause an immediate, intense, physical reaction—particularly anger, disgust, or impulsivity.
- Tourette syndrome is a neurological condition involving repetitive, involuntary movements and vocalizations (tics). Issues may be overresponsivity to certain stimuli; craving intense self-harmful stimuli; and vision and hearing problems.

For these and other overlapping conditions, a multidisciplinary approach combining auditory retraining, counseling, and a sensory-enriched life are among treatments that bring some relief.

BEING A CHILD

Naturally, the growing child will push away certain foods, ignore a grown-up's instructions, crave action when being quiet is expected, break toys, stumble and fall. Unless these behaviors constantly make the child and everyone around him miserable, do not worry. Let's remember a universal condition that often looks like SPD: behaving like a typical kid!

4

Understanding Sensory Processing—and What Can Go Amiss

Understanding basic information about sensory processing and SPD is important. You need to know about the senses, the developmental stages of sensory processing through which a young child normally progresses, and what happens when sensory processing does not go according to Mother Nature's plan.

The Senses

Our senses give us the information we need to function in the world. Their first job is to help us survive. Their second job, after they assure us that we are safe, is to help us learn how to be active, social creatures.

The senses receive information from stimuli both outside and inside our bodies. Every move we make, every bite we eat, every object we touch, produces sensations. When we engage in any activity, we use most of the senses at the same time. The convergence of sensations—especially touch, body position, movement, sight, sound, and smell—is called integration. This process is key and tells us on the spot what is going on, where and when in our environment or body it is happening, why it matters, and how we must use or respond to the instantaneous sensory messages.

The more important the activity, the more senses we use. That is why we use all our senses simultaneously for two very important human activities: eating and procreating.

Sometimes our senses inform us that something in our environment does not feel right; we sense that we are in danger and so we respond defensively. For instance, should we feel a tarantula creeping down our neck, we would protect ourselves with a fight-or-flight response. Withdrawing from too much stimulation or from stimulation of the wrong kind is natural.

Sometimes our senses inform us that all is well; we feel safe and satisfied and seek more of the same stimuli. For example, we are so pleased with the taste of one chocolate-covered raisin that we eat a handful.

Sometimes, when we get bored, we go looking for more stimulation. For example, when we have mastered a skill, like skating in a straight line, we attempt a more complicated move, like a figure eight.

To do their job well, so that we respond appropriately, the senses must work together. A well-balanced brain that is nourished with many sensations operates well, and when our brain operates smoothly, so do we.

We have more senses than many people realize. The ancient Greek philosopher Aristotle said that we have five senses. Today, some folks who study the senses claim that we have twenty-one . . . or fifty-three! For our purposes, eight are enough, with some sensations occurring on the outside of our bodies and some inside.

THE EXTERNAL SENSES

The sensory systems that receive messages coming from outside our body and beyond are sometimes called the external or environmental senses. Think of them as public senses; lots of people can see the same moon and hear the same thunder.

Everyone is familiar with five senses:

- The tactile sense tells us about touch messages received through the skin (see chapter 5).
- The visual and auditory senses tell us about sight and sound messages received through the eyes and ears. (See chapters 8 and 9.)
- The olfactory and gustatory senses tell us about smell and taste messages received through the nose and mouth. (These senses are not explored in this book.)

THE EXTERNAL (ENVIRONMENTAL) SENSES

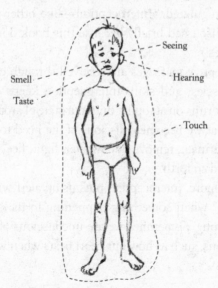

Seeing

Smell

Hearing

Taste

Touch

We are conscious of our external senses and we have some control over them. We can squint to avoid the glaring sun or scrutinize a photograph of all the third-graders to find our child. We can cover our ears to screen out a jackhammer or listen for birdcalls. We can jam our hands into pockets or touch a petal with one fingertip. As we mature, our brains refine our external senses so that we can respond in self-protective and satisfying ways to the world around us.

THE INTERNAL SENSES

Less familiar are the internal senses—sometimes called the so-matosensory (*somato* means body in Greek) or body-centered senses. Think of them as private senses; only one person knows what is going on inside you. Three internal senses are always with us, and we cannot block them.

One of these internal senses is interoception, providing information about our emotional and body states and keeping us self-regulated. (Interoception—like other fascinating topics—is discussed briefly because this book does not have enough pages!)

Interoceptive messages are received through our internal organs, muscles, and skin. Interoception keeps our bodies humming. It runs on autopilot until our state of arousal reaches the point that we become conscious of the need to act, i.e., to eat, drink, urinate, remove our sweater, fight, flee, freeze, hug and kiss, and so forth.

Furthermore, interoception puts us on alert with a strong "gut feeling" when something happening to us is very odd, scary, or wrong. Sometimes we are unconscious of interocep-tive sensations, such as how our heart beats when we are calm.

THE INTERNAL (BODY-CENTERED) SENSES

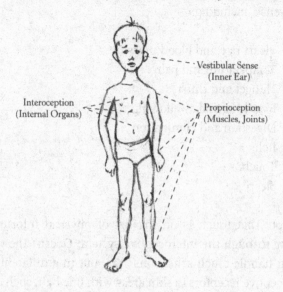

Interoception (Internal Organs)

Vestibular Sense (Inner Ear)

Proprioception (Muscles, Joints)

Other times we are quite conscious of these sensations. When our heart beats fast, and we get "all shook up" because we are fired up for the home team, excited about birthday presents, scared about making a speech, or sexually aroused, we know it.

How Interoception Affects a Child's Behavior

A Typical Child	A Child with SPD
After recess, Joe, eleven, is thirsty and hot. He hangs up his jacket, goes to the washroom, rinses his hands and wrists, splashes water on his face, and takes a long drink. Refreshed inside and out, he is ready to settle down for math.	After recess, Don, eleven, is unaware that he is dehydrated and hot. Removing his coat or drinking water does not occur to him. Disoriented, he straggles to his desk. The math lesson begins while Don, flushed and sweaty, stares out the window.

Interoception provides physical information about one's body sense, including:

- Heart rate and blood pressure
- Temperature and pain
- Hunger and thirst
- Breathing and swallowing
- Digestion and elimination
- Itch
- Touch
- Sleep

Note that touch is on the list of physical information coming through the interoceptive system. Doesn't the tactile system handle touch sensations? Yes, but in a different way. Interoceptive receptors in skin areas with fine hair, such as the arm or calf, are stimulated by messages about social touch, such as a mother's caress. Meanwhile, tactile receptors in hairless skin areas, such as the palm and fingers, are stimulated by messages about physical qualities of objects, such as the weight, texture, and shape of an orange.[1]

Interoception provides emotional information about one's sense of self, including:

- State of arousal
- Empathy
- Mood
- Love and hate
- Motivation
- Laughing and crying
- Intuition
- Nervousness

According to Cara Koscinski, OTD, the current state of our body, both physically and emotionally, affects us as we go about our business of daily living. In her book *Interoception: How I Feel*, she says, "When we are asked to focus on demands of work, family, and school, we may be forced to ignore how our body truly feels in order to perform functions and tasks. [Those with SPD] may not feel the physical and psychological cues such as hunger, thirst, failure, and stress, [or they] may not be able to ignore and suppress interoceptive information, and thus behavior is affected."[2]

In addition to interoception, two other internal senses give us crucial information:

- The vestibular sense provides information about the position of our head in relation to the surface of the earth, the movement of our head through space, and our balance. Sensations come through the inner ear. (See chapter 6.)
- The proprioceptive sense, or proprioception, provides information about our body position and movement of body parts. Sensations come through muscles, joints, and ligaments. (See chapter 7.)

Of all these senses, Dr. Ayres highlighted the importance of the tactile, vestibular, and proprioceptive senses that provide the sense of oneself in the world. Fundamental for functioning, these three senses lay the groundwork for a child's healthy development. When they operate automatically and efficiently, the child can then turn his eyes, ears, and attention to the external environment.

Typically, a child is born with his sensory apparatus intact, ready to begin his lifelong work of sensory processing and integration.

What Is Sensory Processing?

Sensory processing is the neurological procedure of organizing the information we take in from our bodies and the world around us for use in daily life. Sensory processing is dynamic, ceaseless, and cyclical. It occurs in the nervous system, which consists of a spinal cord, a brain, and 86 billion neurons.[3]

According to Dr. Ayres, "Over 80% of the nervous system is involved in processing or organizing sensory input, and thus the brain is primarily a sensory processing machine."[4] When our brain efficiently processes sensations, we respond automatically with adaptive responses that help us master our environment. Adaptive responses are actions or thoughts that help us meet new challenges and learn new lessons. When we feel safe and need not put every effort into staying alive, we can use sensations to get on with the everyday human occupations of moving, learning, playing, working, and enjoying relationships with others.

Sensory processing involves reception, detection, integration, modulation, discrimination, postural responses, and praxis. These processes are simultaneous. Here are the basics, in an extremely simplified discussion of an extremely complex process.

RECEPTION AND DETECTION

One process is sensory reception. Every minute of every day, millions of sensations are received in the peripheral nervous system (PNS)—the nervous system outside the spinal cord and brain, where nerves begin and end. ("Peripheral" literally means "carried around," i.e., away from the center.) Sensations from the skin, muscles, ears, eyes, mouth, and nose travel through the PNS to the CNS (central nervous system). Imagine the incoming sensations saying, "Knock, knock! Here we are!"

In the process of detection, the CNS notices these sensory messages. The brain says, "Come in, all you sensations! I can see (hear, touch, smell, etc.) you!"

INTEGRATION

Integration is the continuous part of the process whereby sensations from one or more sensory systems connect in the brain. "Meet the gang!" the brain says to the various sensations. "Touch, team up with vision. Hearing, connect with movement." The greater the number of sensory systems involved, the more accurate and multidimensional the information will be—and the more efficient the person's adaptive response will be.

MODULATION

Another component of sensory processing is modulation. This is the term used to describe the brain's regulation of sensory input. Modulation instantly adjusts and balances the flow of sensory information into the CNS. The sensory systems need to work in tandem to keep us in sync.

Incoming sensations activate sensory receptors in a process called excitation. Excitation promotes connections between sensory input and behavioral output. Excitation is alerting. "Pay attention!" the sensations insist.

Most of the time, we do pay attention to meaningful sensory messages. If moving rhythmically in a rocking chair is calming, our brain gives us the go-ahead to continue. If spinning in circles makes us feel sick, our brain usually directs us to stop.

Sensations advising us that we are in danger are highly significant. We are hardwired to pay attention to our danger signals in order to defend ourselves. Like all creatures, the human baby is born with sensory wariness, which he needs for survival. When potentially harmful stimuli touch him in some way, his nervous system says, "Uh-oh! Quick! Do something!"

The majority of sensations, however, are irrelevant. In a process called inhibition, our brain allows us to filter out useless information and focus on what matters at the moment. Without inhibition, we would be extremely distractible, giving full attention to every sensation, useful or not. For instance, it is unnecessary to respond to the sensation of air on our skin or to a shift in balance when we take a step, so we learn to ignore the messages. The brain says, "Settle down. That's nothing to get excited about. Do not even think about it."

Some messages are unimportant now, although they initially grabbed our attention. After a while, when we have become accustomed to familiar messages, habituation occurs. This process tunes sensations out because they are no longer extraordinary. At first, we sense the tautness of the seat belt or the tartness of the lemon drop—and then get used to it.

Habituation does not occur readily for everyone. A process called sensitization may be the norm for sensory-sensitive people. Their brain interprets stimuli as important, unfamiliar, or harmful, even if the stimuli are unimportant, familiar, or benign. Quicker and longer than other people, they notice sensations and are bothered or distracted by them. Always, the seat belt feels too tight and the lemon drop tastes too tart.

How Modulation Affects a Child's Behavior

A Child with Typical Modulation	A Child with SPD
During recess, Marian, seven, plays jacks and ignores the cold pavement because the game interests her. Her hands are cold, though, so she does not play well. The first time she fails to scoop up the jacks, she's disappointed. The second time, she's annoyed. The third time, she's thoroughly frustrated. She says, "I'm going to jump rope." Jumping for a few minutes warms her up and makes her feel better. After recess, Marian returns to her classroom and is calm and attentive until lunchtime.	Beth, seven, is playing jacks. She cannot concentrate because the cold pavement distracts her. On her first two turns, she has trouble scooping up the jacks. Beth tries again, but her hands are too stiff. Suddenly, she explodes and screams, "I hate jacks!" She jumps to her feet, kicks the jacks into the grass, and leans against the building, crying uncontrollably. Unhappy all morning, she cannot calm down to attend to the reading lesson, and she refuses to eat lunch.

Here is an example to illustrate modulation: Imagine turning on the gas jet to warm the teakettle. At first, you turn the dial a bit too far, too fast, and the gas leaps high. If you keep the dial there, the water will quickly come to a boil. But if you twist the dial back to inhibit the gas, the gas will calm down and heat the water at a moderate pace. You have modulated the amount and intensity of the fire.

When excitation and inhibition are balanced, we can make smooth transitions from one state to another. Thus, we can switch gears from inattention to attention, from sulks to smiles, from drowsiness to alertness, and from relaxation to readiness for action. Modulation determines how efficiently we self-regulate, in every aspect of our lives.

SENSORY DISCRIMINATION

Another aspect of sensory processing is discrimination, which is the awareness of sensory messages and the ability to discern their similarities and differences within a particular sense. Discrimination has to do with the temporal and spatial characteristics of sensations—that is, with time and space.

Say you are on the beach, playing Frisbee with your child. The Frisbee flies through the air. With good sensory discrimination, you perceive it coming toward you, judge how fast it is approaching and where it is in space, and run at the right pace to the right place to catch it. "Aha!" the brain says as it processes all that Frisbee information. "I know what this means and just how to respond!"

Sensory discrimination allows us to perceive:

- Qualities of sensations—How fast am I moving? Is my voice loud? Have I chewed this carrot enough? Are my shoes tight? Is this bucket heavy?
- Similarities of sensations—Does "four" rhyme with "door" . . . or with "five"? Will this jigsaw piece fit into that empty space? Is my right arm stretched as high as my left arm? Does this dog feel like my cat?
- Differences among sensations—Do I hear someone saying "bag" or "bad"? Does this pear look ripe and yummy or overripe and yucky? Which train is moving—the one I am on or the one on the adjacent track? Is this towel cold or wet?

Sensory discrimination develops with neurological maturation. As a child matures, he responds less self-protectively to every sensation and becomes more discriminating about what is happening in his body and the environment. He learns to use sensations for organized behavior. For instance, when Granny arrives at the door, the child runs for a hug because integrated sensations about whom he has touched, what he has seen and heard, and how he has moved through space teach him how to respond.

Please note: Discrimination should take precedence over defensiveness in everyday situations. Of course, at any age, a person can always revert to defensiveness when a true threat occurs, for this capability diminishes but does not disappear.

The chart below gives a general picture of how this shift occurs as the child develops.

How Sensory Discrimination Takes Precedence over Sensory Defensiveness as Children Mature

Child's Age	Growing Importance of Discrimination
Infant: Defensiveness is weightier.	Discriminative / DEFENSIVE
Toddler: Defensiveness and discrimination level off.	Defensive / Discriminative
Kindergartner: Discrimination is weightier.	Defensive / DISCRIMINATIVE

SENSORY-BASED MOTOR SKILLS

In a nanosecond, the CNS receives, detects, integrates, modulates, and discriminates incoming sensory messages. The end result of sensory processing is when the brain sends outgoing messages that prepare the person to do something. Immediately, the brain says, "Okay, let's move!" (Or, "Let's act! Let's not act! Let's think! Let's pay attention! Let's talk, cry, or giggle!")

For instance, when motor output goes to the arms, legs, eyes, and other body parts, it prepares the child to move in a satisfying way that encourages her to do more and to do it better. Motor output involves postural responses and praxis.

Postural Responses

Efficient sensory processing is necessary for normal movement. Equipped with the sensory information he needs, the child has good postural responses and bilateral coordination.

Postural responses extend the child's trunk, neck, and head upward, against the pull of gravity. His equilibrium and bilateral coordination allow him to experiment with different movements and positions. The child can get into and stay in a stable position. He can get into an unstable position, too, such as leaning over to retrieve a dropped pencil, and then regain his balance.

With firm muscle tone, he bends and straightens his muscles to stretch and reach. He grasps, turns, and releases objects such as spoons and doorknobs. He gets on a swing, holds on, and stays put. He enjoys different kinds of weight-bearing movement, such as crawling and doing push-ups. Changing positions smoothly, he shifts his weight from foot to foot or rotates body parts, swirling his arms around his torso like a flag on a pole.

The child maintains his balance and upright position when

standing or sitting. He uses both sides of the body together to catch a ball, watch a bird fly, and jump with both feet. He uses one side alone to kick a ball, and by the age of four or five, he draws with a preferred hand.

Good postural responses contribute to the child's confidence that he can control his body and master new challenges.

Praxis

How do you learn to jump, hop, skip, type, or flip pancakes? How do you get to Carnegie Hall? Praxis, praxis, praxis!

Praxis is based partly on efficient, unconscious sensory processing and partly on conscious thought. It is a broad term denoting coordinated and voluntary action. Praxis is the process of:

1) Ideating, or conceptualizing, an unfamiliar and complicated action involving several steps,
2) Organizing one's body to carry out the plan (motor planning), and
3) Executing, or carrying out, the plan—or at least making some progress.

Praxis permits us to do what we need and want to do as we go about our occupations of daily living. Thanks to praxis, we can pump on a swing and pump gas, write on paper and paint at an easel, grind pepper and punch an elevator button, suck sesame seeds from our teeth and whistle "Happy Birthday."

No child is born with praxis. Praxis is a learned skill. The child develops it over time as she touches and explores objects and learns to move her body in different ways. Each time she rehearses ordinary actions such as zipping her jacket and organizing her backpack, her motor planning skills improve.

Mastering one motor skill leads to trying another that is more challenging. The more the child does, the more she can do. For instance, after gaining confidence on a jungle gym, a child may use her skills to climb a tree or hang upside down from the monkey bars. This is an example of adaptive behavior.

Sensory Processing Working as It Should

In a nutshell, sensory processing involves input, organization, and output. Sensory input is the neurological process of receiving messages from receptors inside and on the surface of the body. In the next step, the brain organizes the sensations. In the motor output part of the process, the brain sends out instructions to the body so the person can do what she wants to do—run, play, climb, talk, eat, sleep, and so forth. As the person engages in all these human activities, the movement of the body and the doing of the activity lead to more sensory input through the sensory receptors and more feedback to the brain. The illustration on page 79 shows this cycle.

Here is how sensory processing works: Suppose you are sitting on the couch, reading your mail. You pay no attention to the upholstery touching your skin, or the car passing by outside, or the position of your hands. These sensory messages are irrelevant and you do not need to respond to them.

Then your child plops down beside you and says, "I love you." Simultaneously, your senses of sight, hearing, touch, movement, and body position (and maybe smell, too) are stimulated. Sensory receptors throughout your peripheral nervous system take in all this information and sweep it into your CNS. The information zooms to your brain.

THE PROCESS OF SENSORY INPUT, ORGANIZATION, MOTOR OUTPUT, AND CONTINUAL FEEDBACK[5]

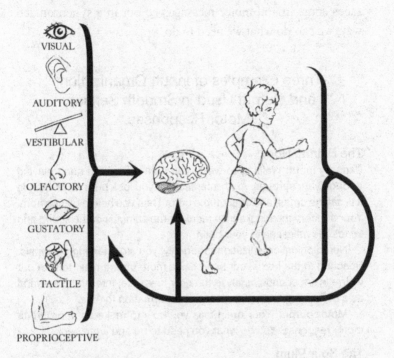

Now these sensory messages are relevant. Swiftly, your brain organizes them and then sends messages back out so you can produce a sensory-motor response.

You respond with language: "I love you, too."

You respond with emotion: a gush of affection.

And, because you know where you are and where your child is, you know how much time it will take to get to her. Anticipating how much force to use for a "feel good" hug, you respond with movement. You drop the mail, lean over, open your arms, and embrace your child.

No one part of the CNS works alone. Messages must go back and forth from one part to another. When sensory messages come in and motor messages go out in a synchronized way, we can do what we need to do.

Three Examples of Input, Organization, and Output Used in Smooth Sensory Motor Responses

The Blaring Horn

Sensory input: Walking to work, you hum along to a song playing through your earbuds. At an intersection, you look both ways, decide it is safe to cross, and step off the curb. Then you hear a blaring horn. Your auditory (hearing) sense receives the stimulus of the sound and sends the message to your brain.

Neurological organization: Suddenly, you stop hearing the music. Reacting to the horn, your brain has a more urgent task: to filter out all irrelevant sounds, analyze the new message, interpret the sound as a danger signal, and organize the information for use.

Motor output: Your brain tells you how to make an appropriate motor response. You do what you need to do and jump back.

The Sour Plum

Sensory input: You see a plum that looks juicy, ripe, and sweet. You bite into it and discover that your expectation was wrong; it is sour. Your gustatory (taste) sense sends the message to your brain.

Neurological organization: Your brain reacts, interprets "sour" as harmful, and organizes the sensory message for use.

Motor output: Your brain tells the muscles in your mouth how to respond. You spit out the morsel and tell yourself to check more carefully the next time.

The Tilting Chair

Sensory input: Seaside, you lower yourself into a folding aluminum chair. The chair's back legs plunge into the sand. Unexpectedly, you tip backward. Your vestibular (movement) sense sends the message to your brain.

Neurological organization: Your brain reacts and analyzes this loss of equilibrium.

Motor output: Your brain instructs you to protect yourself. Your core muscles contract, your head cranes forward, and your hands grab the armrests. You regain your balance without tumbling backward into the sand.

The more efficient our brain is at processing sensory input, the more effective our behavioral output will be. The more effective our output, the more feedback we receive to help us take in new sensory information and continue life-sustaining, never-ending sensory processing.

The Typical Development of Sensory Processing in Infants and Children

Becoming functional is a developmental process. It evolves as the maturing child builds his sense of self.

Dr. Ayres used a diagram to show the four levels of sensory development.[6] Her concept could be compared to a child's block construction. At first, the little child pushes blocks around on one level. Eventually, he figures out how to add a second level to the first. Then he adds a third level, and a fourth.

Sensory processing builds the same way. Each level rests on the building blocks laid down before. Just as the top level of the child's block building needs support, so his readiness for complex skills rests on the foundation of the tactile, vestibular, and proprioceptive senses. (See appendix B for a discussion of the four levels.)

By the time a child is ready for preschool, the blocks for complex skill development should be in place. What are these blocks?

- Ability to modulate touch sensations through the skin, especially unexpected, light touch, and to discriminate among the physical properties of objects by touching them (tactile sense),
- Ability to adjust one's body to changes in gravity, and to feel comfortable moving through space (vestibular sense),

A VARIATION OF DR. AYRES'S FOUR LEVELS OF SENSORY INTEGRATION

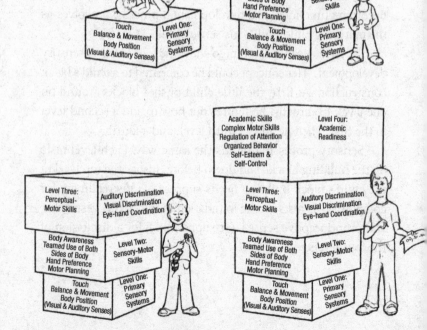

- Ability to be aware of one's body parts (proprioceptive sense),
- Ability to use the two sides of the body in a cooperative manner (bilateral coordination), and
- Ability to interact successfully with the physical environment; to think of, plan, organize, and carry out a sequence of unfamiliar actions; to do what one needs and wants to do (praxis).

Every child has an appetite for sensory nourishment. Inner drive, or self-motivation, urges him to participate actively in experiences that promote sensory processing. In daily life, he explores the environment, tries new activities, and strives to meet increasingly complex challenges. Mastering each new challenge makes him feel successful, and success gives him the confidence to forge ahead.

So, What About Sensory Processing *Differences*?

This chapter, thus far, has been about typical sensory processing. What about sensory processing *differences*?

Differences are to be expected, because everyone responds to sensations in his or her own way. Some like it hot/noisy/turbulent/peppery/bright, and some like it cool/quiet/gentle/unflavored/shady, and so forth.

At one end of the continuum, the highly developed sensory processing abilities of gifted children give them huge advantages. At the other end of the continuum, the underdeveloped sensory processing abilities of out-of-sync children present them with huge challenges. Sometimes a child will be both gifted, say in academics or music, and also out of sync, say in writing or sports; this child is described as "2e," or "twice exceptional." (To learn about twice-exceptionality, see www .withunderstandingcomescalm.com.)

The differences that are the focus of this book cause a child to have difficulty interacting effectively at school and in the community. Sensory stimulation may cause challenges in the child's movement, emotions, attention, or adaptive responses.

Having SPD does *not* imply brain damage or disease, but rather what Dr. Ayres called "indigestion" of the brain, or a "traffic jam in the brain."[7] Here is what may happen:

- The child's central nervous system may not receive or detect sensory information.
- The brain may not integrate, modulate, organize, and discriminate sensory messages efficiently.
- The disorganized brain may send out inaccurate messages to direct the child's actions. Deprived of the accurate feedback he needs to respond purposefully, he may have problems in looking and listening, paying attention, interacting with people and objects, processing new information, remembering, and learning.

Pinpointing a person's specific type of SPD matters greatly in order to determine appropriate treatment and help him "come to the table," be part of the family or classroom team, and engage in active, meaningful play.

The categories of sensory modulation differences, sensory discrimination differences, and sensory-based motor differences were mentioned in chapter 2. They are explained more fully here.

SENSORY MODULATION DIFFERENCES

Differences in sensory modulation are common among children with SPD. The problem is with timing in the CNS. Inhibition must be timed just right to balance excitation so that simultaneous sensory messages can be synchronized.

What happens when a child's nervous system cannot synchronize sensations effectively? The child may be overresponsive, underresponsive, sensory craving, or have a combination of these.

Sensory Overresponsivity: The Sensory Avoider—"Oh, No!"
The most frequently seen type of a sensory modulation problem is overresponsivity to sensations in one or several systems. Overresponsivity—or "hypersensitivity"—to touches and sounds is common.

An overresponsive child with quick or intense inhibition has a low threshold for sensations, whether they are meaningful or meaningless, positive or negative. He is the teakettle with the gas turned up too high. Sensations "pour on the heat," activating all his receptors. He responds to them all, roiling and boiling, bubbling over. He needs help to simmer down.

The child's brain cannot inhibit sensations efficiently. He may be quite distractible because he is paying attention to all stimuli, even if the stimuli are not useful. Overaroused and unable to screen the irrelevant from the relevant, he seeks to defend himself from most sensations. (This behavior is sometimes called sensory defensiveness.) He may respond as if they were irritating, annoying, or even threatening.

Most people alert to a novel sensory experience—say to a light touch or a lump in the mashed potatoes—and then shrug it off, but this child cannot let it go. Instead of responding with a typical "Oh, what's that?" he may respond with "Oh, no! Don't do this to me!" Most people respond to a scary situation—say a bumblebee or angry shouts—with a fight, flight, freeze, or fright response, eventually calming down, but this sensory avoider goes to extremes.

How does his fight, flight, freeze, or fright response play out? If "fight" is his modus operandi, he responds with vigorous resistance or hostility. He may be negative and defiant, lashing out.

If "flight" is his manner, he makes an aversive response. An aversive response is a feeling of revulsion and repugnance toward a sensation, accompanied by an intense desire to avoid or turn away from it. The child may actively withdraw, fleeing from the sensations by running away, jumping back, hiding under the table, climbing on furniture, or trying to claw his way out, desperate to get away from the perceived threats.

Or he may "flee" by withdrawing passively, simply avoiding the people and objects that distress him. He never gets close to them or he walks away. Often, adults think he avoids messy play and merry-go-rounds because "those just aren't his thing." In fact, he may yearn to participate in the activities his peers enjoy, but just can't.

If "freeze" is his style, he may stop in his tracks, unable to move, speak, or even breathe.

If "fright" is his way, then his world is a scary place. Everything may make him crumple and cry. Or he may be fearful and cautious, closing out unfamiliar people and situations.

However possible, he will avoid sensations, particularly touch and movement experiences, because he cannot tolerate them. He may be distressed by changes in routine, loud noises, and crowded settings. He may misinterpret a casual touch as a life-threatening blow or feel that he will fall off the face of the earth if he is nudged. "Close connections between sensory processing and emotional regulation explain why children with SPD can respond in ways that seem so over the top," say Brock Eide, MD, and Fernette Eide, MD, in their book *The Mislabeled Child*. They "frequently respond to powerful environmental stimuli as if they were in mortal peril: They truly believe that they are."[8]

For the child with overresponsivity, meltdowns are common. A meltdown, according to clinical psychologist Jed Baker, PhD, author of *No More Meltdowns*, is an escalating negative emotional reaction, usually to sensory overload.[9] Screaming, writhing, and deeply sobbing, the child falls to pieces. Unlike a temper tantrum that a neurotypical child performs publicly to get someone's attention and that vanishes when he gets what he wants, a meltdown may be a private, lonely, scary event for the child with SPD. He melts down not to get attention but because he cannot cope with the excessive sensory stimulation.

Meltdowns may happen several times a day, be emotional and loud, and last a long time, perhaps hours. Their frequency, intensity, and duration may be "off the scale," going far, far beyond other children's responses to the same situation.

Once they begin, meltdowns cannot be stopped until they have run their course. The best approach is to stop them before they begin. OTs and therapists like Dr. Baker can help parents and teachers learn ways to anticipate the triggers, keep their own emotions in check, find calming strategies, and create a plan to prevent future meltdowns. Sarah Wayland, PhD, a parenting coach,[10] says that you may gradually notice that the meltdowns' duration gets shorter. Then their frequency lessens. Then their intensity softens. While they may not disappear completely, to your great relief they will eventually become manageable for you and the child.

Another issue may be difficulty understanding gestural communication. The child may overreact to nonverbal cues, such as laughter or raised eyebrows, and respond with anxiety or hostility. He may be extremely sensitive to someone else's displeasure, even if the displeasure is not directed toward him. Relating to and communicating with family members, classmates, and other people in the child's world—the skill called social pragmatics—may be a big challenge.

Sensory Underresponsivity: The Sensory Straggler— "Wait, What?"

Underresponsivity—or "hyposensitivity"—to sensations is another subtype of sensory modulation differences.

An underresponsive child with slow inhibition has a high threshold for sensations. She is the teakettle with the gas turned too low; she is not receiving enough heat to get activated. She needs help to light her fire.

The child reacts less intensely to sensations than do typically developing children. The sensory straggler needs a lot of stimulation just to achieve ordinary arousal or alertness. Her response to the world is "Wait, what?"

Sensory modulation has many dimensions. One child's sensory underresponsivity may cause her to be withdrawn and difficult to engage. She may be interested only in her interior life and her own body.

On a different dimensional path, another sensory straggler may be so talented and creative that he does not notice sensory stimuli because he is self-absorbed and preoccupied with intellectual pursuits. He may ignore life around him, including his own body, and appear to live in his own universe. He may seem passive, lacking initiative, and unable to get going. He may tire easily and seem sleepy, and as a baby, he may have slept and slept and slept.

Also, the underresponsive child may eat and eat and eat, perhaps unaware that he is full. (Give him water, soup, or fresh fruit to fill him up before meals, and serve smaller portions.) He may chew on inedible objects, such as shirt cuffs and toys, to get sensory information through his mouth. (Offer chewing gum and search online for "sensory chewies" to satisfy his oral-motor urges.)

The sensory straggler may miss cues that other children catch easily. He may bump into desks and people because he does not perceive them in time to move aside. He may hurt himself because he does not register "hot" or "sharp" as painful sensations. The child may have trouble understanding gestural communication. He may misinterpret nonverbal cues and respond slowly to unspoken messages. He may not "read" other people's facial expressions and body language. He may not laugh at a clown's antics, may not comprehend that the teacher is beckoning the children to go indoors, and may not respond to a person's frown or an animal's growl.

Sensory Craving: The Sensory Craver—"More, More!"

The sensory-craving child hungers for more stimulation than other children and never seems to get enough. He is the tea-kettle that needs the gas turned on full blast. "More, more, more!" he cries. He is addicted to certain stimuli. He may be a "toucher and feeler" and a "bumper and crasher." His brain and body are telling him that he must act, but he often acts in a disorganized way.

He likes to burp and flatulate, talk and hum. He may chew on his fingers and shirt cuffs and collar for extra input.

He craves movement and seeks vigorous experiences, such as spinning for exceptionally long times on the tire swing. Often, he will not feel dizzy. He may get into upside-down positions, with his head hanging over the mattress. He is a climber—on the monkey bars at the playground and on the bookshelf, the windowsill, and the car roof. Another characteristic of the sensory craver is that he may seek one kind of sensation but pay scant attention to others.

Busy TV screens may attract him, as may strobe lights, loud noises, and places with plenty of action, such as football games and car races. Seeking strong odors that others find objectionable, he may sniff food, people, and objects. He may crave spicy foods, tart lemons, and red-hot candy.

This child is often a risk taker and a daredevil and may also have poor impulse control. No wonder others frequently look upon him as a troublemaker.

Sensory Combination: The Sensory Fluctuator— "I Love This, I Hate That"

Another sensory modulation difference is a combination of over- and underresponsivity as the child's brain rapidly shifts back and forth. Fluctuating, or mixed, responsivity may cause differing behaviors with similar sensations, depending on the kind of stimuli, the time, the place, what she ate, how much sleep she had, the arousal state of her body, and other factors. Her CNS is undecided, saying, "I love this, I hate that."

Sometimes the sensory fluctuator will seem to be in sync and sometimes she won't. She may cringe from messy play *and* crave movement *and* be unaware of smells. She may seek intense sensory experiences, such as spinning, but be unable to tolerate them—or crave them on Tuesday and avoid them on Friday. She may dislike loud noises or being touched passively, yet use a loud voice and touch everything in sight actively. How common it is to be not all one way!

The child has great difficulty functioning in daily life. She is not on an even keel and becomes easily upset. Once upset, she may have difficulty recovering. Her attention span for things she enjoys may be excellent until certain sensations get in her way. She may be well regulated, feeling safe and in control at home, but uncertain and out of control at school, or vice versa. The need to feel in control of people, objects, and experiences is a major issue for the child who does not feel in control of herself.

Her behavior bewilders the adults who care for her. This child is particularly challenging to raise and to teach, because knowing how to support her feels like guesswork.

SENSORY DISCRIMINATION DIFFERENCES

The Sensory Jumbler—"What Does That Mean?"
The child with sensory discrimination differences has difficulty differentiating among and between stimuli within one sense. Is the bathwater warm enough or too hot? Has he chewed the peanut sufficiently or is it not yet ready to swallow? What is it that hurts—an earache or toothache or stomachache?

The child's CNS inaccurately processes sensations, so he is unable to use the information to make purposeful, adaptive responses and function throughout the day. He misgauges the importance of objects and experiences. He may not "get" sensory messages that others use to protect themselves from injury, to learn about their environment, and to relate successfully to other people.

The child often has significant difficulty with visual-spatial tasks. He may be unable to judge where objects and people are in space and may miss important visual cues on the page and in social interactions. He often has auditory discrimination problems, too. These cause him to be easily confused by similar-sounding words or by verbal instructions.

This sensory jumbler may have poor body awareness, falling frequently and having difficulty catching himself. He uses inappropriate force when using pencils, manipulating toys, and playing with other children. He breaks pencils, struggles to fit Legos together, and bumps into people and things because he does not notice them.

The sensory jumbler often is overresponsive to certain sensations. Overresponsivity to, say, tactile sensations means that he may avoid touching mud, shampoo, buttons, and corn on the cob. Thus, he will have difficulty discriminating these items' physical qualities, because to know many things, one must handle them. Just looking at them is not enough.

When the sensory jumbler has challenges with touch, movement, and body position, he often has dyspraxia, too. That is no surprise, as praxis requires sensory discrimination about how one's body works.

SENSORY-BASED MOTOR DIFFERENCES

In addition to modulation and discrimination differences, a child with SPD may have sensory-based motor differences that affect how she moves.

Postural Challenges: The Sensory Slumper—
"Don't Want To"

Postural issues cause the child to have difficulty with moving or stabilizing her body. She may have low muscle tone and be "loose and floppy," resulting in poor posture. She slouches while sitting or standing and slumps over the desk and dining room table. This droopy child is besieged by the "gravity monster," a descriptive term coined by the Australian OT and songwriter Genevieve Jereb. The reason may be the inefficient sensory processing of vestibular and proprioceptive sensations about where her body is in space and what it is doing.

According to Dr. Ayres, "The major symptoms manifested by children with this type of dysfunction . . . are related to the fact that man is a bilateral and symmetrical being."[11] When a child has not developed a sense of two-sidedness, postural challenges may interfere with nature's plan, which is to keep upright and ready to spring into action, using both sides of the body together or separately as needed.

The child may have a problem with bilateral integration, the neurological process of connecting sensations from both sides of the body. The result is poor bilateral coordination, the ability to use both sides of the body together. For instance, she may struggle to gallop, skip, or pedal a bicycle.

She may have difficulties positioning her body and maintaining her equilibrium. Getting into different positions, such as kneeling or stretching to her tiptoes, without tipping over may also be a challenge.

Often the child will have poor ocular (eye movement) control, affecting binocularity—the use of both eyes together as a team. This will hinder depth perception, body movement, motor planning, and reaching for objects. Difficulty crossing the midline—i.e., using the eye, hand, or foot of one side of the body in the space of the other eye, hand, or foot—may interfere with her ease in painting a horizon at the easel or swinging a baseball bat.

Keeping up with her peers wears her out. Her grasp on doorknobs and faucets, toys and lunchboxes, is weak. When she sits on the floor, her legs are often in the W position, with her knees pointing forward and feet splayed to the side for added stability.

Flexing and extending her muscles, shifting her weight from one foot to the other, twisting her body around while planted on two feet, moving like animals, and so forth are movement activities that we expect children to enjoy. For the sensory slumper, they are often too daunting.

Dyspraxia: The Sensory Fumbler—"I Can't Do That"

Dyspraxia is the second type of sensory-based motor differences. Dyspraxia refers to disruption in sensory processing and motor planning in children who are still developing.

Dyspraxia causes children to be clumsy and ineffective in their actions. They cannot organize their bodies to move. They reach for a stair tread or a water bottle and they miss—a problem called motor overshoot. Dr. Ayres says that "these children may have normal intelligence and muscles. The problem is in the 'bridge' between their intellect and their muscles."[12] For some reason, accurate information about touch, movement, and body position cannot cross that bridge from the brain to the body, so the child does not "get it" and cannot use it. (Many examples of how SPD leads to dyspraxia are in the next chapters.)

Possible Causes of SPD

Challenging sensory processing differences may be caused by:

1) A genetic or hereditary predisposition, often the case if the child's parent, sibling, or other close relative has some SPD

2) Prenatal circumstances, including:
- chemicals, medications, or toxins like lead poisoning that the fetus absorbs
- the mother's drug or alcohol abuse or smoking
- maternal stress
- unpreventable pregnancy complications, such as a virus, a chronic illness, great emotional stress, or a problem with the placenta
- multiple births (e.g., twins or triplets)

3) Prematurity or low birth weight

4) Birth trauma, perhaps due to an emergency cesarean section, a lack of oxygen, or surgery soon after birth

5) Postnatal circumstances, including:
- environmental pollutants
- limited opportunities to move, play, and interact with others
- lengthy hospitalization
- early life stress, such as caregiving deprivation at home or in an institution like a poorly run orphanage; poverty; food scarcity; and other forms of social/emotional neglect that result in insufficient stimulation to early neurodevelopment
- adverse childhood experiences, such as sexual abuse, warfare, and other physical threats that cause excessive stimulation

6) Unknown reasons

Exciting research is answering many questions about SPD. Dr. Ayres's explorations, decades ago, laid the foundation for current research, such as sophisticated quantitative or functional brain imaging studies that demonstrate anatomical differences in the brains of out-of-sync children. Research on the gut microbiome suggests that the health of the gut affects the health of the brain. As scientists make clearer distinctions among those with sensory issues, increased knowledge about the roots of SPD will lead to the most effective interventions.

Six Important Caveats

In this book, you will find many checklists of characteristics of children with SPD. You will also find numerous examples of out-of-sync behavior that illustrate the various ways SPD plays out at home and school. You may say, "Eureka! This is my child, to a tee!" On the other hand, you may say, "This is definitely not my child, because my child does not have all these symptoms." Perhaps your child is somewhere in between.

As you read along, please remember the following caveats:

1) The child with SPD does not exhibit every characteristic mentioned in this book. Nobody has them all.

2) The child with SPD usually has difficulties in more than one sense, but she may have a concentration of problems in one system. If so, she will not necessarily exhibit every characteristic of that category. For example, the child with vestibular differences may have poor balance but good muscle tone; the child with tactile differences may find light touch intolerable but be a good eater.

3) The child may be both overresponsive and underresponsive in one sensory system, or may be overresponsive to one kind of sensation and underresponsive to another, or may respond differently to the same stimulus depending on the time and context, fluctuating back and forth. Yesterday, after a long recess, he may

have coped well with a fire alarm; today, when recess is canceled, he may have a meltdown when a door clicks shut. Context makes a huge difference.

4) Categories of SPD are not always clear-cut and often overlap. Sensory overresponsivity and sensory under-responsivity, for instance, often look like and merge with sensory discrimination differences and dyspraxia.

5) The child may exhibit characteristics of SPD yet have another condition altogether. For example, the child who typically withdraws from being touched may seem to have tactile overresponsivity but instead may have a childhood anxiety disorder or may have been physically abused.

6) Everyone has some sensory processing problems now and then, because no one is well regulated all the time. All kinds of stimuli can temporarily disrupt functioning of the brain, either by too much or too little sensory stimulation.

Comparison of Typical Sensory Processing and SPD

	Typical Sensory Processing	SPD
What:	The ability to take in sensory information from one's body and the environment, to organize this information, and to use it to function in daily life.	The ineffective processing of tactile, vestibular, and/or proprioceptive sensations. The person may have difficulty with other basic senses, too.
Where:	Occurs in the CNS (nerves, spinal cord, and brain), in a well-balanced, reciprocal process.	Occurs in the CNS, where the flow between sensory input and motor output is disrupted.
Why:	To enable a person to survive, to make sense of the world, and to interact with the environment in meaningful ways.	Neuronal connections in the CNS are ineffective.
How:	Happens automatically as the person takes in sensations through sensory receptors in the skin, the inner ear, the muscles and joints, and the eyes, ears, mouth, and nose.	Sensory neurons do not send effective messages in to the CNS, and/or motor neurons do not send effective messages out to the body for adaptive behavioral responses.
When:	Begins in utero, developing through childhood, with most functions established by adolescence.	Occurs before, during, or shortly after birth.

5

How to Tell if Your Child Has SPD in the Tactile Sense

Three Kindergartners at Circle Time

The kindergartners are gathering for circle time. In the center of the rug, Miss Baker has arranged a variety of squashes: acorn, butternut, pattypan, pumpkin, summer, and zucchini.

Most of the children sit down on their individual carpet squares. Robert, however, stands aside and waits until the others are seated. Then he gingerly picks up his carpet square and moves it toward the wall. He pulls two plastic dinosaurs from his pocket and grips one in each hand. Finally, he sits down, as far as possible from Lena, his nearest neighbor.

Patrick finds his carpet square, but instead of sitting, he makes a crash landing, sprawling facedown on the rug. He spreads his arms and legs and swishes them on the rug, shouting, "Look! I'm a windshield wiper!"

Miss Baker says, "Please sit up in your own space, Patrick."

He sits up and begins to wrestle with another boy until Miss Baker says, "Please keep your hands to yourself, Patrick."

Eventually, circle time begins. Miss Baker passes each squash around the circle, so the children can get a feel for them.

Patrick squeezes every squash when he gets his hands on it. He rolls the summer squash between his hands and rubs it down his legs. He licks the acorn squash and bites the zucchini.

Miss Baker reminds him, "Just use your hands, not your mouth. And please pass the squash to Lena. It is her turn."

Lena, however, is not paying attention. She gazes out the window. When Patrick flings each squash into her lap, she looks down in surprise. Without examining the squashes, she passes them quickly to Robert.

But Robert refuses to touch the vegetables. When Lena offers him the first squash, he jabs his dinosaurs toward her face.

Lena recoils and drops the squash. Having figured that Robert is not receptive, she places the subsequent samples in front of him.

Using his dinosaurs, Robert pushes each squash away.

Miss Baker lines up the squashes in the center of the rug. She says, "Now, look at the squashes. What can you tell me about them?"

Several children volunteer their observations: "The pumpkin is heavy." "The zucchini is smooth." "The pattypan has a bumpy edge."

Miss Baker says, "You are good observers! What about you, Lena? Do you have something to add?"

Lena hesitates. Then she says, "I see six."

"True!" says Miss Baker. "Anything else?"

"Nothing," Lena says.

Miss Baker turns to Robert and says, "How about you?"

Robert says, "This is boring."

"This isn't boring!" Patrick bellows. He lunges forward, scoops all the squashes into a pile, and rolls on top of them. "This is fun!"

Miss Baker extricates the squashes from Patrick and says, "Let's put the squashes away now and sing a song. Then it is time for free play in the classroom."

Circle time comes to a close.

ATYPICAL PATTERNS OF BEHAVIOR

To the casual observer, Robert, Patrick, and Lena may seem like typical kindergartners. It is easy to look at their behavior and say, "That is just the way they are." But if we look closer, we may notice atypical patterns of behavior.

Touching and being touched distress Robert. He avoids being near the other children and defends himself with his dinosaurs. Handling his carpet square is unpleasant. He refuses to touch the squashes with his hands.

Touching and being touched delight Patrick. He uses his whole body to feel the rug. He tackles another child. He man-handles, mouths, and rolls on the squashes.

Touching objects to learn about them is not Lena's forte. Giving scant attention to the squashes, she does not perceive whether they are heavy or light, big or small, bumpy or smooth. Her only observation is about their quantity, not their quality.

These children may appear to be very different, but they have something in common: an identifiable problem with the tactile sense.

On the next pages you will learn how the tactile sense is supposed to function, followed by an explanation of the types of SPD that affect Robert, Patrick, and Lena.

The Smoothly Functioning Tactile Sense

The tactile system, or sense of touch, plays a major part in determining physical, mental, and emotional human behavior. Every one of us, from infancy onward, needs constant tactile stimulation to keep us organized and functioning.

We get tactile information through sensory receiving cells—called receptors—in our skin, from head to toe. Touch sensations of light touch, deep pressure, skin stretch, vibration, movement, temperature, and pain activate tactile receptors.

Receptors are dense and sensitive in hairless body parts—fingertips, palms, soles, eyelids, lips, and tongue tip. Receptors in some hair follicles—eyelashes, head hair, and hair around the genitals—are also very sensitive, detecting sensations before they touch the skin. Fewer receptors are in areas covered with fine hair where tactile information is less vitally important, such as the arms, legs, and torso.

While we think of tactile information as coming primarily from the skin, some tactile sensations are internal. Messages about muscle contraction and joint compression through the proprioceptive system (see chapter 7) and messages about our lungs, heart, and bladder through the interoceptive system (see pages 66–68) tell us what is going in inside. This is another example of how the senses are integrated.

We are always actively touching or passively being touched by something—other people, furniture, clothes, spoons. Even if we are stark naked, our feet still touch the ground and the air touches our skin.

When we are comfortable in our own skins, we develop a positive sense of self and of our place in the world. According to Dr. Ayres, "Touch is one of the senses that is especially involved in the ongoing process contributing to perception of other types of sensation. Touch has been one of the predominating senses throughout evolution, is a predominant sensation at birth, and probably continues to be more critical to human function throughout life than is generally recognized."[1]

This huge sensory system connects us to the environment around us and bonds us to others, starting when we first nestle at our mother's breast, skin to skin. It gives us essential information for body awareness, motor planning, visual discrimination, language, academic learning, emotional security, and social skills.

TWO COMPONENTS: DEFENSIVE ("OKAY!" OR "UH-OH!") AND DISCRIMINATIVE ("AHA!")

Two components make up the tactile sense. First is the protective (or defensive) system. Its purpose is to alert us to potentially harmful—or healthful—stimuli. Tactile receptors for this protective system are fast-adapting, responding instantly to light touch.

Sometimes a light touch is alarming, such as a mosquito alighting on our skin. "Uh-oh!" our nervous system tells us. We respond negatively, for self-preservation. Sometimes a light touch is charming, such as a lover's gentle caress, and our nervous system says, "Okay!" We respond positively, for preservation of the species!

Ordinarily, modulation of touch sensations improves as we interact with other people and objects. We learn to inhibit sensations that do not matter and to tolerate trifling touches that would have irritated us in infancy. Of course, when a stranger gets too close, we shrink; when a lash gets in our eye, we blink. But usually, we ignore light touch sensations because they do not grab our attention the way deep pain or extremes in temperature do.

Knowing *that* we are touching something actively or that we are being touched passively is important, of course. Equally important is knowing *what* we are touching or what is touching us.

The second component of the tactile sense teaches us to discriminate just what kind of touch we are feeling. Deep touch, or "touch pressure," is the stimulus that causes the receptors to respond. Slow-adapting receptors provide information about Mommy's smooth cheek, Daddy's rough stubble, the shape of a Lego brick, crunchy granola in the mouth, and bumpy gravel underfoot.

Through discriminative touch, we gain conscious insights, intuition, and knowledge about the world. Where have we felt this touch before? What could that touch signify? And what should we do about it? With the capability to remember and interpret the meaning of touches, we gradually develop tactile discrimination.

"Aha!" the nervous system says, telling us:

- That we are touching something or that something is touching us,
- Where on our body the touch occurs,
- Whether the touch is light or deep, intense or slight,
- How quickly we became aware of it,

- How long we have been feeling it,
- How to perceive the attributes of the object, such as its size, shape, weight, density, temperature, and texture, and
- What the object may be.

As you read on, you will understand why a smoothly functioning tactile system is necessary to function normally, and how differences in tactile processing can get in a child's way.

The Out-of-Sync Tactile Sense

SPD can interfere with the way a child organizes and uses tactile sensations perceived through the skin. The child often has difficulty touching, and being touched by, objects and people. He may have one or more problems with modulation, discrimination, or sensory-based motor skills as he goes through the day.

SENSORY MODULATION DIFFERENCES

Tactile Overresponsivity—"Oh, No!"
The child with overresponsivity to touch has the tendency to respond negatively and emotionally to unexpected, light touch sensations. The child will respond this way not only to actual touch but also to the anticipation of being touched. Perceiving most touch sensations to be uncomfortable, scary, or outright terrifying, he overresponds with a fight, flight, fright, or freeze response.

He may wrestle in your arms as you try to dress or lift him. He may wriggle out of his clothes or car seat. He may kick, punch, or scream at anyone who comes too close for comfort.

How Tactile Overresponsivity
Affects a Child's Behavior

A Child with Typical Modulation	A Child with SPD
Getting ready for preschool, Isaac, three, tolerates having his father brush his hair and wash his face. He does not enjoy this experience, but he can adapt to it and can recover immediately. His maturing neurological system allows him to suppress a fight-or-flight response.	Getting ready for preschool, Will, three, flinches when his father tries to brush his hair and wash his face. He pushes his father away and cries, "You're hurting me!" Defensiveness still rules his reactions to touch, so he produces an infantile fight-or-flight response. He is upset all during breakfast.

The child may flee from contact with finger paints, pets, and people. He may find the touch of unfamiliar people to be intolerable. Or he may withdraw passively by simply avoiding the objects and people that distress him. He never gets close to them, or he walks away.

He may be later than other children to develop self-help skills. He may be afraid and start to cry when he must remove his clothes and take a bath. He may stop dead in his tracks and not know what to do when his cuffs get wet at the sink.

All children need touch information to learn about the world. So how does the child with tactile defensiveness get this information? By touching!

Parents are often mystified when they learn that their child has tactile overresponsivity. They protest, "But he often asks for hugs and back rubs. He usually carries something in his hands. How can you say he has a problem with touch?"

The answer is the type of touch that the child avoids or seeks. The child typically avoids passive, unexpected light touch, such as a gentle kiss. A kiss is irritating, and the child may try to rub it off. While the child avoids light touch, he not only accepts but also craves deep touch, like a bear hug. A hug provides firm touch and deep pressure, which feels wonderful and actually helps suppress sensitivity to light touch.

While the child may long for the hug, he may reject the hugger unless the hugger is on his "okay" list. A likely okay person is a parent or another predictable individual whom the child trusts. People on his "not okay" list may be classmates, babysitters, relatives, and even loving grandparents, to their great sorrow.

This child needs touch information more than children with a well-regulated tactile sense who get it just by waking up in the morning and going through the day. To get the stimulation his brain needs, he may actively, repeatedly touch those surfaces and textures that provide soothing and comforting tactile experiences. For example, he may cling to a beloved stuffed animal or blanket. He may also hold objects such as a stick or a toy in his hand. He may mouth toys. Perhaps these objects help him defend himself from the unexpected touch sensations abounding in the environment.

Tactile Underresponsivity—"Wait, What?"

The underresponsive child seems not to notice touch, whether it is soothing or painful. Instead of murmuring, "Mmm!" when his mother cradles him, he may not seem to respond, or he may respond slowly, as if to say, "Wait, what is happening?" Instead of crying, "Ouch!" when he stubs his toe, he seems to say, "Didn't notice."

Unlike the ever-alert, overresponsive child, the sensory straggler may not respond to touch effectively enough to do a good job of self-protection. In fact, he may seem unaware of touch altogether, unless the touch is very intense.

How Underresponsivity
Affects a Child's Behavior

A Child with Typical Modulation	A Child with SPD
Randy, six, falls off his bicycle, scraping his knees. He runs inside and tearfully tells his babysitter that he had a bad accident. She bandages his wounds and soothes him. Eventually, he stops crying, although he hobbles around the house and complains for a little while. As soon as his friend comes to play, he forgets about his discomfort.	Georgio, six, falls off his bicycle. He scrapes both knees but pays little attention to his injuries. He remounts his bike and continues to ride. When his babysitter notices his wounds and tries to clean them, he brushes her off. "It doesn't hurt," he says.

Sensory Craving—"More!"

All children need abundant sensations to learn about the world. The sensory craver's difference is in needing more deep pressure and more skin contact than most. He may touch and feel everything in sight, running his hands over furniture and walls, and handling items that other children understand are "no-nos." Even if an object is inappropriate to handle, such as a fragile dish or a hot candle, he's "gotta touch" it.

Intensely and impulsively, he may seek to touch certain surfaces and textures that are uncomfortable to others, rubbing his hands over rough tree bark and walking barefoot on gravel. He crams his mouth with food. He gets too close to other people, bumping, pawing, and touching them, although they tell him this is unwelcome. Messy play is his true love. He will look for and find puddles, mud, clay, glue, and paint. The more the merrier.

The sensory craver frequently gets in trouble for his insistent, persistent tactile explorations. His constant wallowing in

How Sensory Craving Affects a Child's Behavior

A Child with Typical Modulation	A Child with SPD
The kindergarten teacher gathers the children around a table covered with a plastic cloth. She spurts a mound of shaving cream in front of each child. Viggo, five, enjoys finger painting in the cream. He smears it around his table space and writes his name in it. When Bryce begins to bother him, he shouts, "Stop!" and moves back. He rinses his hands and finds a puzzle to do at a table far away from Bryce.	Bryce, five, adores playing with shaving cream, the teacher's smart substitute for finger paint. He smears the cream over his hands, arms, throat, and face. He begins to smear Viggo, who says, "Stop! You'll get in trouble!" Bryce turns back to the table, spreading shaving cream into other children's territories. They object and the teacher comes over to intervene. He could play here all day, but his behavior is getting in everyone else's way.

messy materials ruins his clothes, trashes the classroom, and repels the people around him. Of course, his motivation is not to infuriate them but to get the sensory input his nervous system needs. Of course, most people do not understand his behavior. And, of course, the child is incapable of explaining his cravings, so everyone around him gets upset and tells him he is being bad.

Therapy can help this child's nervous system to modulate touch sensations. At home and school, an approach may be to provide him with a lot of safe, appropriate, fun, and easy tactile activities. (See *The Out-of-Sync Child Has Fun* for specific suggestions.)

Sensory Combination—"I Love This, I Hate That"

The sensory fluctuator may have overresponsivity and underresponsivity to sensations, like two sides of a coin. One minute, he may truly love an experience such as having his hair brushed or being cuddled, and the next minute he may hate it. He may shriek with alarm when someone touches his arm, yet be indifferent to a broken collarbone. He may love jumping on the mattress and hate getting a back rub. This, but not that! That, not this!

How a Sensory Combination Affects a Child's Behavior

A Child with Typical Modulation	A Child with SPD
Peter, ten, and his friend Cody decide to kick a can all the way home instead of riding the bus. Invigorated from the walk, the boys are now in the kitchen, twisting dough to make pretzels. Peter does this often and is comfortable getting his hands dirty; he likes to mold and sculpt the dough into animal and people shapes.	Today Cody enjoys handling the sticky pretzel dough after walking to Peter's instead of taking the bus. Everything with Peter is fun. Then Peter's sister starts to play the saxophone. The squeaky blasts irritate Cody, and suddenly the fun is over. He can't tolerate the dough on his hands another second. He runs to the sink, scrubs his hands, and rushes out without saying thank you or goodbye.

TACTILE DISCRIMINATION DIFFERENCES

"What Does That Mean?"

The child with discrimination differences may have difficulty paying attention to the physical attributes of objects and people. If he has a modulation problem, his central nervous system is otherwise occupied. For instance, if he is a sensory avoider, his hands may "live" in his pockets or he may keep his fingers curled to protect his sensitive palms. If he is a sensory craver, he may handle—or mishandle—everything in sight without discrimination.

When sensory modulation is out of sync, then the child's discriminative system may not arise to "take charge." (The child

with poor tactile discrimination often has tactile overresponsivity, but this is not always the case.) With inefficient or immature discrimination, the child will have difficulty using his
tactile sense for increasingly complex purposes, such as learning at school. Even when he has met building blocks or three-
ring binders before, he needs to touch and handle them
repeatedly to learn about their weight, texture, and shape.
"Huh?" he seems to say. "What does this mean?"

The child may seem out of touch with his hands, using
them as if they were unfamiliar appendages. He may be unable
to point a finger toward the book he wants or to button a coat
without looking at what he is doing. He may have difficulty
learning new manual skills, exploring materials and equipment, using classroom tools, and performing ordinary tasks. If
he gets a bee sting, he may not perceive where it is on his body,
when it began to hurt, or whether the pain is increasing or
lessening.

How Tactile Discrimination Affects a Child's Behavior

A Typical Child	A Child with SPD
Kindergartner Ellie is making a "harp" by pulling rubber bands over a cigar box. Tactile discrimination helps her grasp differences among the rubber bands. She chooses several with various attributes: big and small, skinny and fat, tight and loose. She stretches them over the box and arranges them carefully so they do not overlap. By strumming or plucking, she produces a variety of pleasing sounds.	Patsy, five, grabs a huge handful of rubber bands, but she has trouble knowing which ones are more or less flexible than others. They all seem the same to her, because her tactile discrimination is inefficient. She struggles to stretch one rubber band around the cigar box and then gives up. Problems with modulation, discrimination, and dyspraxia get in her way.

How the Tactile Sense
Affects Everyday Skills

In addition to helping us to protect ourselves, to discriminate among objects, and to accomplish what we set out to do, the tactile sense gives us information that is necessary for many kinds of everyday skills:

- Body awareness (or body percept)
- Praxis (motor planning)
- Visual discrimination
- Language
- Academic learning
- Emotional security
- Social skills

BODY AWARENESS (BODY PERCEPT)

The tactile sense, along with the proprioceptive sense, affects a person's subconscious awareness of individual body parts and how the body parts relate to one another and to the surrounding environment. With good tactile discrimination, a child develops body awareness (body percept), which is like a map of the body, and can then move purposefully and easily. The child has a sense of where he is and what he is doing.

The child with tactile processing differences may lack good body awareness. He is uncomfortable using his body in his environment because moving means touching. He has difficulty orienting his limbs in order to get dressed. He would rather stand in a corner than risk mingling with an unpredictable group. Shifting his position may even make him conscious of how uncomfortable he is in his clothes. Better to stand very, very still, his central nervous system tells him, and avoid it all.

How Body Awareness Affects a Child's Behavior

A Typical Child	A Child with SPD
In his third-grade music class, James is enjoying the song "Head and Shoulders, Knees and Toes." He likes it when the tempo speeds up, so that tapping the right body parts at the right time gets harder. Recess is after music, and James slips into his jacket, zips it up, pulls on his gloves, and heads outdoors.	Roger slumps in the back row, scowling. He hates the "Head and Shoulders" song. It goes too fast, and he gets confused with his body parts. Before recess, he concentrates on getting into his coat, still a challenge. Gloves are uncomfortable, so he shuffles outdoors with his hands stuck in his pockets.

PRAXIS (MOTOR PLANNING)

Each new sequence of movements requires praxis, or motor planning. Certainly, the first time a child climbs a jungle gym, threads a belt through loops, or says "Lollapalooza," he must plan his movements with conscious effort. With practice, he can do these actions successfully because he has integrated tactile sensations, such as the feel of the jungle gym rungs under his feet and hands.

The child who feels uncomfortable in his own skin may have dyspraxia, sometimes called poor motor planning. He may move awkwardly and have difficulty planning and organizing his movements. Thus, he may shun the very activities that would improve his praxis.

For instance, if he dislikes how the monkey bars feel, he may not try to hang from them or practice the skill of traveling

How Praxis (Motor Planning) Affects a Child's Behavior

A Typical Child	A Child with Dyspraxia
Charley, four, arises and puts on blue jeans and a new belt, managing to buckle it all by himself. He runs downstairs. He steadies his grapefruit with one hand and spoons it with the other. Ready for school, he climbs into the car and fastens his seat belt. Arriving at school, he unsnaps his seat belt and jumps out. On the blacktop, he spots a new tricycle. It is larger than the trikes he has ridden before, but he figures out how to mount it. He stretches his feet and arms to reach the pedals and handles. He takes it for a test drive, getting a feel for its new requirements.	Lars, four, arises slowly. He ignores the clothes his mother has set out; they're too hard to put on. He struggles into his favorite pants with the elasticized waist. He goes downstairs carefully: right foot, then left, on each step. He jabs a spoon at his grapefruit, and the dish skitters across the table. When it is time to go, he maneuvers himself into the car and waits for his mother to buckle him in. Arriving at school, he needs help to unbuckle the seat belt. He inches out of the car. On the blacktop, Lars heads for an old familiar tricycle. While the other kids ride in circles around him, he sits there, dangling his feet.

beneath them, one hand after the other. If touching a dandelion makes him uneasy, he may not reach to pick it. The less he does, the less he can do. In a world where "use it or lose it" is a fact of life, this child may be at a loss.

Gross-Motor Control

Praxis is necessary for two broad categories of movement, one of which is gross-motor control. Like the superhighway, this is the smooth coordination of the large, or proximal, muscles, which are closest to the body core. Gross-muscle control allows a child to bend, lift, twist, stretch, move his body from one place to another by creeping or running, and maneuver his hands and feet.

The child with tactile (and proprioceptive) processing differences may be out of touch with his body and with objects in his world. His gross-motor skills may be delayed, making it very difficult to learn, move, and play in meaningful ways.

How Gross-Motor Control Affects a Child's Behavior

A Typical Child	A Child with SPD
Gwen, ten, enjoys the fast-moving "over and under" game. One person holds a ball over her head and passes it to the next person, who takes the ball, bends forward, thrusts it through her legs, and passes it to the next. Moving is fun!	For Kim, ten, playing "over and under" is hard. Her movements are slow and awkward. The ball feels uncomfortable in her hands, and sometimes she drops it. When she slows down or interrupts the game, the other kids get angry. Movement games are no fun at all.

Fine-Motor Control

Praxis is necessary for another category of movement: fine-motor skills, like the byroads, which a child usually refines after establishing gross-motor skills. Fine-motor control governs the precise use of small muscles in the fingers and hands, in the toes, and in the tongue, lips, and muscles of the mouth.

Because the child with tactile processing differences often curls his hands into loose fists or jams them in his pockets to avoid touch sensations, he has difficulty manipulating ordinary tools such as eating utensils, scissors, crayons, and pencils. So much of the school day revolves around writing and other fine-motor tasks that a problem with these skills may be extremely discouraging for the older child.

This child frequently has poor self-help skills, is a messy eater, and may also have poor articulation and immature language skills. He may use more gestures than words to communicate because the fine-motor control of his tongue and lips is inadequate.

How Fine-Motor Control Affects a Child's Behavior

A Typical Child	A Child with Tactile Dysfunction
Today is woodworking day for Alex's preschool class. Alex sorts through the woodbin, chooses two pieces, and hammers them together to make an airplane. He takes it outside and experiments with different ways to hold and throw it. At dinner, he explains in detail how he constructed his lovely airplane and how well it flies. Alex has good praxis.	Roy, four, wants to construct an airplane. He is not sure how to begin, so the teacher hands him two wood pieces. He has trouble holding the hammer, so the teacher helps him. His airplane looks pretty good. Outside, he stands and holds it until it is time to go home. At dinner, his father asks what he did at school. Unable to express his thoughts, Roy holds up his lovely airplane for his father to see. Roy is dyspraxic.

VISUAL DISCRIMINATION

The tactile system plays an important part in the development of visual discrimination—the way the brain interprets what the eyes see. By touching objects, a child stores memories of their characteristics and relationships to one another. Looking at a rain puddle, for instance, he perceives that it is wet, cool, and

How Tactile Processing
Affects a Child's Visual Discrimination

A Typical Child	A Child with SPD
The teacher hands each kindergartner a plastic shape. Each shape has different attributes. It is big or small; red, yellow, or blue; round, square, or rectangular. Then the teacher lays similar shapes on the rug and asks the children to tell her which shape on the floor matches the one in their hands. Joye knows the answer right away because she has handled many objects in her five years. She places her small red square next to its mate.	The teacher hands Chrissy, five, a big yellow rectangle, and Chrissy drops it into her lap. When her turn comes to match her shape with one on the floor, Chrissy is uncertain about its size and shape. She knows her colors, though. She makes a guess and puts her big yellow rectangle next to a small yellow square. A classmate points out her error, and the teacher asks him to show Chrissy how to make a correct match.

fun to splash in, even without touching it, because he has touched puddles before.

Normally, a young child touches what he looks at and looks at what he touches. Many experiences touching objects and people are the basis for visual discrimination.

When a child's brain mismanages touch stimuli, however, he cannot integrate tactile and visual messages. Basic information eludes him about how things appear to feel. He looks but does not understand what he sees.

LANGUAGE

The tactile sense, in a way, leads us to language. Babies depend on touch to make contact with the world. Expanding their contacts as they move around and touch things, young children absorb others' commentaries about what they are doing.

"That's a daisy. Touch it gently."

"Pull hard on that wagon. Pull, pull!"

"Give me your foot and I'll put on your shoe."

"Where is the ball? It is under the couch. Get the ball. Throw the ball to Daddy."

"Whoops! You fell down, head over heels! That was scary. Come here; I will brush you off and make it all better."

Words become associated with actions, body parts, objects, places, people, and feelings. Thus, children learn verbs, nouns, names, prepositions, adjectives, adverbs, and labels for emotions.

How Tactile Processing Affects a Child's Language

A Typical Child	A Child with SPD
Jeff's eighth-grade cooking class made delicious tacos last week. Today the teacher asks the students to write down the recipe to test their memory about the various steps and processes involved. Jeff writes, "Warm taco shells in preheated oven. Grate cheese. Shred lettuce. Mince chipotle chilies. Chop cilantro. Dice tomatoes and peppers. Sauté ground beef or turkey. Drain fat. Peel and slice onion, and sauté. Spread mixture on taco shells. Arrange condiments in bowls so guests can choose what they like." Et cetera.	Gavin, thirteen, enjoys eating and thought taking a cooking class as an elective would be easy, but preparing the food is hard. Dyspraxia and tactile discrimination differences cause him to fumble with the taco ingredients, measuring spoons, and knives. He jumbles everything together. Now he is supposed to write down the recipe but is vague about the manual tasks involved and the words to describe them. He wishes he could prove to the teacher that his motivation to do well is high . . . but how? He writes, "Cook meat. Cut vegetables. Serve."

When the out-of-sync child's tactile experiences are limited, so are his opportunities to develop language. In addition, the child with poor tactile awareness in his mouth, lips, tongue, and jaw may have a sensory-based motor problem called oral apraxia, which affects his ability to produce and sequence sounds necessary for speech.

ACADEMIC LEARNING

Tactile processing has a big impact on a child's ability to learn at school. Many objects require hands-on manipulation: art and science materials, math manipulatives, keyboards, basketballs, chalk, pencils, and paper. Taking pleasure in tactile experiences leads to exploring new materials and building a base of knowledge that will continue throughout a lifetime.

Tactile differences prevent a child from learning easily because touch sensations distract him. He may fidget when quiet is expected, complain that others are annoying him, and have trouble settling down for academic tasks.

How the Tactile Sense Affects a Child's Academic Learning

A Typical Child	A Child with SPD
Juan, six, likes science. Today, the teacher brings several caterpillars in a glass jar. Juan knows how it feels to handle caterpillars and asks, "May I hold the one that looks soft and fuzzy?" The teacher offers him the jar. He picks out the fuzzy caterpillar and puts it on his arm. "It tickles!"	Ricardo, six, dislikes science. While the other first-graders talk about the caterpillars, Ricardo averts his gaze. He rejects the teacher's invitation to hold the jar. He squirms in his chair and sits on his hands. He hates creepy bugs.

The child misses out on learning skills requiring the purposeful use of tools such as compasses, forks, and hammers. He misses out on learning about nature because messy, hands-on experiences are intolerable or because he cannot discriminate between an acorn and a chestnut. He misses out on learning problem-solving skills, communication skills, and people skills.

EMOTIONAL SECURITY

With a well-regulated nervous system, we first learn to welcome the touch of the person (usually our mother) who takes care of our basic infantile needs. Cuddling makes us feel safe.

A close physical attachment to one or two primary caregivers sets the stage for all future personal relationships. If we feel cared for and loved, our emotional base is secure, and we learn to reciprocate warm feelings. Furthermore, if we are in touch with our own emotions, we develop empathy for other human beings. Even if we do not like a person, we know he feels pain when he cuts his finger and pleasure when he takes a bath.

Establishing strong attachments can be very difficult for the child with tactile differences. The overresponsive child may withdraw from ordinary affection, while the underresponsive child may not seem to notice it.

Feeling empathy can also be hard. The overresponsive child feels pain or discomfort where others do not; the underresponsive child appears to feel little pain or discomfort where others do. He may be unable to relate well to another person's feelings.

How the Tactile Sense
Affects a Child's Emotional Security

A Typical Child	A Child with SPD
At ten, Mike takes pleasure in going away to Boy Scout camp. He is comfortable in novel settings and likes making new friends. One night the scouts play a creative thinking game: "What would you need on a desert isle?" Mike suggests a bucket to catch rainwater, a sleeping bag, and binoculars—familiar objects that he has handled—as well as someone to talk to. Mike's well-regulated tactile sense gives him emotional security.	Tim, ten, is unhappy at camp. He misses his mother. He depends on her totally and exclusively for emotional support and always wants her nearby. Forming attachments to others is hard because everyone else seems unreliable. When the scouts play the desert isle game, he has no suggestions; all he can think is that he hates the idea of being deserted, hates being a Boy Scout, and hates being away from home.

The child may have difficulty experiencing pleasure, enthusiasm, and joy in his relationships because of his responses to touch. While he needs even more love than others, he invites less. His insecurity in the world puts his emotional well-being at risk, as a child and as an adult.

Indeed, many adult relationships flounder when one partner's tactile processing difference interferes with emotional intimacy. Too little touching makes the other person feel rejected; too much touching makes the other feel disrespected.

Tactile differences may also limit a child's imagination. Fantasy and make-believe may be beyond his scope, and discriminating real from pretend may be hard. He may be a rigid, inflexible thinker.

SOCIAL SKILLS

A well-regulated tactile sense is fundamental for getting along well with others. Building on the primary mother-child bond, we begin to reach out to others, gladly and comfortably touching and being touched. When we enjoy being near people, we learn how to play, one of the unique characteristics of being human. Thus, it becomes possible to develop meaningful human relationships.

When the child responds to physical contact in ways that are incomprehensible to most people, they may turn away. The sensory straggler who does not notice touch will have difficulty in social situations, as will the sensory craver or "bad boy" who tackles others because he seeks deep-touch pressure, and the sensory jumbler, slumper, or fumbler who cannot use touch messages effectively.

The sensory avoider who withdraws from touch has particular problems with socialization. Standoffish behavior sends signals that he is unfriendly and prefers to be left alone. Seeming to reject others, he is rejected in turn. He has difficulty dealing with the give-and-take, rough-and-tumble world of "playground politics."

Children with tactile overresponsivity frequently mature into adults who are "cool characters." They may be cautious, controlled, and inflexible people. They may seem distrustful or judgmental. Their behavior may be considered "touchy"—a funny word for people who avoid touch! Of course, with a select group they can develop social relationships built on shared interests that often do not involve physical interaction.

How the Tactile Sense
Affects a Child's Social Skills

A Typical Child	A Child with SPD
Standing in line to go to the lunchroom, Jake, eight, playfully bumps into Lewis. Lewis bumps him back. Laughing, they collide a few more times until all the third-graders are lined up and ready to go. When the teacher turns her attention to them and raises her eyebrow, the boys regain control and walk peacefully down the hall. Jake's positive reaction to tactile sensations is the foundation of his good social skills.	Curtis, eight, always tries to be last in line so no one is behind him. But today Eli brings up the rear and grazes him as they go down the hall. Overresponding, Curtis punches Eli. Eli punches back. The boys begin to argue, and the teacher pulls them apart. Curtis complains, "Eli started it. It's his fault." Eli says, "I touched him accidentally! He's such a baby." Relating to his peers is hard because Curtis is uneasy when they get near.

Characteristics of Tactile Differences

The following checklists will help you gauge your child's tactile processing differences. As you check recognizable characteristics, you will begin to see emerging patterns that help to explain your child's out-of-sync behavior. Not all characteristics will apply, but many checked boxes suggest that SPD affects your child.

The **sensory avoider with overresponsivity** has differences with passive touch (being touched). He may:

❑ Respond negatively and emotionally to light-touch sensations, exhibiting anxiety, hostility, or aggression. He may withdraw from light touch, scratching or rubbing the place that has been touched. As an infant, he may have rejected cuddling or nursing as a source of pleasure or calming.

❑ Respond negatively and emotionally to the *possibility* of light touch. He may appear irritable or fearful when others are close, as when lining up at school.

❑ Respond negatively and emotionally when approached from the rear, or when touch is out of his field of vision, such as when someone's foot grazes his under a blanket or table.

❑ Show fight-or-flight response when touched on the face, such as having his face washed.

❑ Show fight-or-flight response to hair displacement, such as having his hair brushed or receiving a haircut, shampoo, or stroke on the head. A high wind or even a breeze can raise his hairs, literally "rubbing him the wrong way" or "ruffling his feathers."

❑ Become upset in weather with rain, wind, or gnats.

❑ Be excessively ticklish.

❑ Overrespond to physically painful experiences, making a "big deal" over a minor scrape or a splinter. The child may remember and talk about such experiences for days. He may be a hypochondriac.

❑ Respond similarly to dissimilar touch sensations. A raindrop on his skin may cause as adverse a response as a thorn.

❑ Strongly resist being touched by a barber, dentist, nurse, or pediatrician.

❑ Exhibit behavior that seems stubborn, rigid, inflexible, willful, verbally or physically pushy, or otherwise "difficult" for no apparent reason, when it is actually an aversive response to tactile stimuli.

❏ Rebuff friendly or affectionate pats and caresses, especially if the person touching is not a parent or familiar person. The child may reject touch altogether from anyone except his mother (or primary caregiver).

❏ Be distracted, inattentive, and fidgety when quiet concentration is expected.

❏ Prefer receiving a hug to a kiss. He may crave the deep-touch pressure of a hug, but try to rub off the irritating light touch of a kiss.

❏ Resist having his fingernails trimmed.

❏ Dislike surprises.

The same **sensory avoider with overresponsivity** also has differences with active touch. He may:

❏ Resist brushing his teeth.

❏ Be a picky eater, preferring certain textures such as crispy or mushy foods. The child may dislike foods with unpredictable lumps, such as tomato sauce or vegetable soup, as well as sticky foods like rice and cake icing.

❏ Refuse to eat hot or cold food.

❏ Be a problem feeder, unable to eat properly.

❏ Avoid giving kisses.

❏ Resist baths, or insist that bathwater be extremely hot or cold.

❏ Curl or protect hands to avoid touch sensations.

❏ Be unusually fastidious, hurrying to wash a tiny bit of dirt off his hands.

❏ Avoid walking barefoot on grass or sand, or wading in water.

❑ Walk on tiptoe to minimize contact with the ground.

❑ Fuss about clothing, such as stiff new clothes, rough textures, shirt collars, turtlenecks, belts, elasticized waists, hats, and scarves.

❑ Fuss about footwear, particularly sock seams. He may refuse to wear socks. He may complain about shoelaces. He may insist upon wearing beach sandals on cold, wet winter days or heavy boots on hot summer days.

❑ Prefer short sleeves and shorts and refuse to wear hats and mittens, even in winter, to avoid the sensation of clothes rubbing on his skin.

❑ Prefer long sleeves and pants and insist on wearing hats and mittens, even in summer, to avoid having his skin exposed.

❑ Avoid touching certain textures or surfaces, like some fabrics, blankets, rugs, or stuffed animals.

❑ Need to touch repeatedly certain surfaces and textures that provide soothing and comforting tactile experiences, such as a favorite blanket.

❑ Withdraw from art, science, music, and physical activities to avoid touch sensations.

❑ Avoid messy play, such as sand, finger paint, paste, glue, mud, and clay, perhaps becoming tearful at the idea.

❑ Stand still or move against the traffic in group activities such as obstacle courses or movement games, keeping constant visual tabs on others.

❑ Treat pets roughly or avoid physical contact with pets.

❑ Arm himself at all times with a stick, toy, rope, or other handheld weapon.

❑ Rationalize verbally, in socially acceptable terms, why he avoids touch sensations, e.g., "My mother told me not to get my hands dirty" or "I'm allergic to mashed potatoes."

❑ Withdraw from a group and resist playing at other children's homes.

❑ Have trouble forming warm attachments with others. Experiencing difficulty in social situations, he may be a loner, with few close friends.

The **sensory straggler with underresponsivity** may show atypical responses to passive and active touch. The child may:

❑ Not notice touch unless it is very intense.

❑ Be unaware of messiness on her face, especially around her mouth and nose, not noticing crumbs on her face or a runny nose.

❑ Be unaware of mussed hair or mulch or sand in hair.

❑ Not notice that clothes are in disarray or that cuffs and socks are wet.

❑ Not notice heat, cold, or changes in temperature indoors or out, often keeping a jacket on even when sweating, or not reaching for a jacket even when shivering.

❑ Show little or no response to pain from scrapes, bruises, cuts, or shots, perhaps shrugging off a broken finger or collarbone.

❑ When barefoot, not complain about the sharp gravel, hot sand, or stubbed toes.

❑ Not react to spicy, peppery, acidic, hot or "mouth-burning" food—or, on the other hand, may crave this kind of food.

❑ Be oblivious to weather conditions with wind, rain, or gnats.

❏ Fail to realize that she has dropped something.

❏ Not move away when leaned on or crowded.

❏ Appear to lack "inner drive" to touch, handle, and explore toys and materials that appeal to most other children.

❏ Require intense tactile stimulation to become engaged in the world around her, but not actively seek it.

❏ Hurt other children or pets during play, seemingly without remorse, but actually not comprehending the pain that others feel.

The **sensory craver** needs extra touch stimuli, both passive and active. The child may:

❏ Ask for tickles or back rubs.

❏ Enjoy vibration or movement that provides strong sensory feedback.

❏ Need to touch and feel everything in sight, e.g., bumping and touching others and running hands over furniture and walls. The child has "gotta touch" items that other children understand are not to be touched.

❏ Rub certain textures over her arms and legs to get light-touch input.

❏ Rub or even bite her own skin excessively.

❏ Constantly twirl hair in fingers.

❏ Frequently remove socks and shoes.

❏ Seem compelled to touch or walk barefoot on certain surfaces and textures that other people find uncomfortable or painful.

❏ Seek certain messy experiences, often for long durations.

❏ Seek very hot or cool room temperature and bathwater.

❑ Have high tolerance for sweltering summer or freezing winter weather.

❑ "Dive" into food, often cramming mouth with food.

❑ Prefer steaming hot, icy cold, extra-spicy, or excessively sweet foods.

❑ Use his mouth to investigate objects, even after the age of two. (The mouth provides more intense information than the hands.)

❑ Show "in your face" behavior, getting very close to others and touching them, even if his touches are unwelcome.

The sensory jumbler with **tactile discrimination differences** may:

❑ Have poor body awareness and not know where his body parts are or how they relate to one another. He may seem "out of touch" with hands, feet, and other body parts, as if they are unfamiliar attachments.

❑ Be unable to identify which body parts have been touched without looking.

❑ Have trouble orienting his arms, hands, legs, and feet to get dressed.

❑ Be unable to identify familiar objects solely through touch, needing the additional help of vision, e.g., when reaching for objects in a pocket, box, or desk.

❑ Be unable to know the difference between similar items he is using, such as a crayon versus a marker.

❑ Be disheveled, with shoes on wrong feet, socks sagging, shoelaces untied, waistband twisted, and shirt untucked.

❑ Avoid initiating tactile experiences, such as picking up toys, materials, and tools that are attractive to others.

❑ Have trouble perceiving the physical properties of objects, such as their texture, shape, size, temperature, or density.

❑ Be fearful in the dark.

❑ Prefer standing to sitting, in order to ensure visual control of his surroundings.

❑ Act silly in the classroom, playing the role of class clown.

❑ Have a limited imagination.

❑ Have a limited vocabulary because of inexperience with touch sensations.

The **sensory fumbler with dyspraxia** may:

❑ Have trouble conceiving of, organizing, and performing activities that involve a sequence of movements, such as cutting, pasting, and coloring; assembling collage pieces or recipe ingredients; applying nail polish; and so forth. Novel experiences as well as familiar activities may be difficult.

❑ Have poor gross-motor control for running, climbing, and jumping.

❑ Have poor eye-hand coordination.

❑ Require visual cues to perform certain motor tasks that other children can do without looking, such as zipping, snapping, buttoning, and unbuttoning clothes.

❑ Put on gloves or socks in unusual ways.

❑ Have poor fine-motor control of his fingers for precise manual tasks, e.g., holding and using eating utensils and classroom tools, such as crayons, scissors, staplers, and hole punchers.

❑ Struggle with handwriting, drawing, completing worksheets, and similar tasks.
❑ Have poor fine-motor control of his toes for walking barefoot or in flip-flops.
❑ Have poor fine-motor control of his mouth muscles for sucking, swallowing, chewing, and speaking.
❑ Be a messy eater.
❑ Have poor self-help skills and not be a self-starter, requiring another person's help to get going.

Your child's primary differences may be with processing tactile sensations. The child may also have difficulty with the internal vestibular and proprioceptive senses, as well as with the external visual and auditory senses.

6

How to Tell if Your Child Has SPD in the Vestibular Sense

Two First-Graders at the Amusement Park

Jason Green is in perpetual motion, but he is not much of a conversationalist. He is a "high motor, low verbal" kid. When he began to talk at three, his few words included "choo, choo" and "toot, toot," for his passion is trains. Jason loves trains so much that his father calls him "our little locomotive."

Kevin Brown, Jason's best buddy, loves trains, too. Kevin behaves not like a train, however, but like a conductor. He is a "low motor, high verbal" child. His mother jokingly calls him "NATO," for "No Action, Talk Only."

When the boys play, Kevin bosses Jason around and Jason cheerfully obeys. Once, Kevin proposed making a train by hitching together a little red wagon, a Big Wheel, and an old tricycle. Jason nodded in agreement. All thumbs, the boys fumbled with rope and finally managed to connect the vehicles. Then Kevin instructed Jason to push the train down his steep driveway so they could watch it plummet into the garage.

Instead of pushing the train, however, Jason clambered into the wagon. "Toot, toot!" he yelled as he plunged down the driveway. Kevin froze. He watched, helpless and horrified, as the train careened out of control.

Jason landed in a heap. He heaved himself up and said, "That was awesome! Totally fantastic! Want to try, Kevin?"

For once, Kevin was speechless.

Today is Jason's sixth birthday, and his parents are taking the boys to the amusement park. Jason loves the Ferris wheel, the merry-go-round, and especially the roller coaster. His idea of heaven is being twirled and tilted in the huge teacup. He never even gets dizzy.

Kevin is less enthusiastic. He has never found amusement parks amusing, because moving fast, high, and around in circles makes him tip over or fall, and the thought frightens him. He likes only the little train that slowly circles the park.

The first attraction the group approaches is the Greased Toboggan. At the top of a slick ramp, riders sit in padded sacks and then slide down. Jason eagerly pulls on his father's sleeve to get his attention and permission.

Mr. Brown and Jason mount the stairs to the top. Jason ascends as fast as he can in his "marking time" fashion. He puts both feet on each step: right first, then left. In his haste, he stumbles twice.

Kevin lingers below with Mrs. Brown, watching. He does not want to slide; he wants to conduct. He raises his arms and shouts, "Go!" each time someone begins to descend. When he lifts his arms, his shoulders rise, too.

Mrs. Brown asks Kevin if he would like to get into a sack with Jason. She points out that lots of people are coming down together in the same sack.

"Oh, no, thank you very much," Kevin says. "You see, I

can't slide down the ramp because I have to tell everyone when to go. I have to make sure that everyone is doing it just right."

Jason and Mr. Brown swoop to the bottom. "That was so awesome!" Jason says. "Now let's go to the roller coaster. That's the most fun of all."

Kevin says, "No, let's go to the train. That's entertaining, and it isn't dangerous for children."

Jason is disappointed but agrees to do whatever his friend wants.

Toot, toot! Chug, chug! Off they go.

ATYPICAL PATTERNS OF BEHAVIOR

Kevin and Jason approach movement experiences very differently. They both show atypical patterns of behavior.

Moving and being moved dismay Kevin. He is uncomfortable on slides and rides that move fast or spin around. He is afraid of heights and prefers to keep his feet on the ground. He relies on his precocious verbal skills to maintain control. Overresponsive to most vestibular sensations, Kevin is intolerant of movement and has gravitational insecurity (see pages 142–43).

In contrast, moving and being moved thrill Jason. Constantly and impulsively, he seeks fast-moving and spinning activities, but he does not get dizzy. Jason is addicted to moving, always craving more, but his movements are disorganized and immature.

In addition to modulation differences, both boys have sensory-based motor differences. Kevin has dyspraxia, which interferes with carrying out his complex plan to make a train. On top of that, he has postural challenges, which make it hard to isolate his movements to raise just one arm without raising the other arm and his shoulders as well.

Jason, too, fumbles with the rope and stumbles up the stairs because of dyspraxia and poor bilateral coordination. Jason also has language problems. To communicate, he often uses gestures such as nodding his head or tugging on his father. He tends to be more talkative, however, after intense vestibular experiences such as sliding down the driveway and riding the Greased Toboggan.

On the next pages you will learn how the vestibular sense typically functions, followed by an explanation of the types of sensory processing differences that derail Kevin and Jason.

The Smoothly Functioning Vestibular Sense

The vestibular system tells us about up and down and whether we are upright or not. It tells us where our heads and bodies are in relation to the earth's surface. It sends sensory messages about balance and movement from the neck, eyes, and body to the CNS for processing and then helps generate muscle tone so we can move smoothly and efficiently.

This sense tells us whether we are moving or standing still, and whether objects are moving or motionless in relation to our body. It also informs us what direction we are going in and how fast we are going. This is extremely useful information should we need to make a fast getaway! Indeed, the fundamental functions of fight, flight, and foraging for food depend on accurate information from the vestibular system. Dr. Ayres writes that the "system has basic survival value at one of the most primitive levels, and such significance is reflected in its role in sensory integration."[1]

The receptors for vestibular sensations are hair cells in the inner ear, which is like a "vestibule" for sensory messages to pass through. The inner-ear receptors work something like a carpenter's level. They register every movement we make and every change in head position—even the most subtle.

Some inner-ear structures receive information about where our head and body are in space when we are motionless, or move slowly, or tilt our head in any linear direction—forward, backward, or to the side. As an example of how this works, stand up in an ordinary bipedal, or two-footed, position. Now close your eyes and tip your head way to the right. With your eyes closed, resume your upright posture. Open your eyes. Are you upright again, where you want to be? Your vestibular system did its job.

Other structures in the inner ear receive information about the direction and speed of our head and body when we move rapidly in space, on the diagonal or in circles. Stand up and turn around in a circle or two. Do you feel a little dizzy? You should. Your vestibular system tells you instantly when you have had enough of this rotary stimulation. You will probably regain your balance in a moment.

What stimulates these inner-ear receptors? Gravity!

According to Dr. Ayres, gravity is "the most constant and universal force in our lives."[2] It rules every move we make.

Throughout evolution, we have been refining our responses to gravitational pull. Our ancient ancestors, the first fish, developed gravity receptors, on either side of their heads, for three purposes:

1) to keep upright,
2) to provide a sense of their own motions so they could move efficiently, and

3) to detect potentially threatening movements of other creatures through the vibrations of ripples in the water.

Millions of years later, we still have gravity receptors to serve the same purposes—except now vibrations come through air rather than water.

In addition to the inner ear, we humans also have outer ears as well as a cerebral cortex, which processes precise vestibular and auditory sensations. These sensations are the vibrations of movement and of sound. (Vibrations stir up all kinds of responses. One day in my music class, I introduced a movement activity by beating a large drum. "Ooooh," said a three-year-old girl, "I can feel that in my bones!" "Me, too," responded a little boy, "and I can even feel it in my penis!")

Nature designed our vestibular receptors to be extremely sensitive. *Indeed, our need to know where we are in relation to the earth is more compelling than our need for food, for tactile comfort, or even for a mother-child bond.*

In her book *Sensory Integration and the Child,* Dr. Ayres explains:

> The vestibular system is the unifying system. It forms the basic relationship of a person to gravity and the physical world. All other types of sensation are processed in reference to this basic vestibular information. The activity in the vestibular system provides a "framework" for the other aspects of our experience. Vestibular input seems to "prime" the entire nervous system to function effectively. When the vestibular system does not function in a consistent and accurate way, the interpretation of other sensations will be inconsistent and inaccurate, and the nervous system will have trouble "getting started."[3]

Whew! What a heavy load! Isn't it astonishing how something you may never have heard of before has such a profound and pervasive influence? As the background for all other senses, the vestibular system gives us a sense of where we stand in the world.

This system, like other sensory systems, has a defensive component. When an infant feels herself falling, she responds to this vestibular sensation as if saying, "Uh-oh!" She extends her arms and legs, groping for something to grab. Her whole body responds in this automatic, self-protective reflex.

As a child grows, her brain integrates reflexive responses in a process called reflex maturation. She learns to discriminate vestibular sensations. She seems to say, "Aha! I am learning to sense what direction I am going in and whether my movement is fast or slow."

Now, when movement sensations help her perceive that she is off center, she learns how to regain her balance. She learns to "stand on her own two feet," in an upright position, against the pull of gravity. She learns to differentiate her body movements so that she can function with an economy of motion.

She can also discriminate among the sounds vibrating in her inner ear, and she learns to listen to what she hears. She can coordinate her own body movements with visual sensations, and she learns to discriminate what she sees.

She learns to enjoy all kinds of movement. One kind is linear movement—back and forth, side to side, or up and down. Slow and low linear movement, which does not challenge gravity, is usually soothing. Parents have known since time immemorial that they can comfort a baby in a rocking chair, in a cradle, or with gentle bounces. In fact, many children (and adults) rock themselves when they are upset, as a kind of tranquilizing self-therapy.

Another kind of movement is rotary—moving around and around. Examples of rotary movement include spinning oneself on a tight axis (e.g., planting one foot on the ground and turning rapidly), riding on a merry-go-round, or swinging high on a long-roped swing. Most children enjoy twirling on a tire swing—even to the point of getting dizzy. Rotary movement stimulates the vestibular system. Usually, it feels good, and that is why it is so much fun!

The Out-of-Sync Vestibular Sense

The child with vestibular dysfunction receives sensations through the inner ear about gravity, balance, and movement through space just like everybody else. Her brain processes the information differently, however, causing vestibular challenges.

The child may not develop the postural responses needed to keep upright. She may never have crawled or crept and may be late learning to walk. She may sprawl on the floor, slump when she sits, and lean her head on her hands when she is at the table.

As she grows, she may be awkward and uncoordinated at playground games. She may fall often and easily, tripping on air when she moves, bumping into furniture, and losing her balance when someone moves her slightly off center.

As eye movements are influenced by the vestibular system, she may have visual problems. She may have inadequate gaze stability and be unable to focus on moving objects or on objects that stay still while she moves. At school, she may become confused when looking up at the board and down to her desk. Reading problems may arise if she hasn't developed brain functions imperative for coordinating left-to-right eye movements.

Vestibular differences may also contribute to difficulty processing language—a great disadvantage in everyday life. The child who misperceives language may struggle to communicate, read, and write.

Many movements provide a calming effect. The out-of-sync child, however, cannot always calm herself because her brain cannot modulate vestibular messages. Difficulty moving smoothly interferes with her behavior, attention, self-esteem, and emotions. The child with an inefficient vestibular system may have modulation, discrimination, and sensory-based motor differences affecting her every move.

SENSORY MODULATION DIFFERENCES

Vestibular Overresponsivity—"Oh, No!"
Vigorous movement, or the possibility of being moved, causes the child with vestibular overresponsivity to respond negatively and emotionally, or to become overexcited.

This modulation difference means that her brain cannot regulate movement sensations the way typical brains can. Her vestibular system is on overload. Particularly when her head or eyes move, her brain is bombarded with sensory stimuli that it cannot organize. Two types of vestibular overresponsivity are intolerance to movement and gravitational insecurity.

Intolerance to Movement—"No, Don't!"
The child who is overresponsive to vestibular sensations may be intolerant of movement. Faulty processing causes aversive

responses: "Oh, no, don't make me move! Moving quickly is too much for me."

How Intolerance to Movement Affects a Child's Behavior

A Typical Child	A Child with SPD
Noah's favorite activities are movement and music. Today, the preschoolers play Noncompetitive Musical Chairs. In this game, no chair is ever taken away. The object is to move around the chairs while the music plays and sit on any seat when the music stops. Everyone plays the whole time; no one is ever "out." When the music starts, Noah jumps up and circles the chairs with the other kids. When the music stops, he slithers into a chair. Once, he lands on another child's lap, but he looks around fast, sees an empty chair, and runs to it. Safe!	Sean, four, dislikes most music and movement activities. Noncompetitive Musical Chairs makes him especially uncomfortable. While the other children run freely around the circle, he inches along, clinging to the seats of the chairs. By the time he has circled the chairs twice, his forehead is sweaty and his stomach is churning. The music finally stops, and Sean sits down with a sigh of relief. When the music resumes, he remains seated.

For her, linear movement is distressing, especially when rapid. Riding in a car—particularly in the back seat—often causes car sickness. She may avoid riding a bicycle, sliding, and swinging at the playground, or just walking down the street.

Rotary movement can be even more distressing. She may become easily dizzy and nauseated on a tire swing. Even watching someone or something spinning can make her feel queasy. Moving in circles may make her head ache and stomach hurt.

If she avoids moving, she may lose the ability to keep up with others. She may become breathless and easily fatigued. Her motor planning skills and coordination may suffer, because she cannot practice them with confidence.

Gravitational Insecurity—"I'm Falling!"

Being connected to the earth is a primal need for survival. The vestibular system tells us where we are in relation to the ground. The trust that we are attached to the earth is called gravitational security.

Usually, a child has inner drive to experiment with gravity. Jumping, swinging, and somersaulting, she can relinquish her grip on the earth for an instant, because she knows she will always return. With this basic sense of stability, she can develop emotional security.

The child with poor modulation may not experience this sense of stability. She feels vulnerable if her feet leave the ground. Lacking a basic sense of belonging to the earth, she has gravitational insecurity, or G.I.

Gravitational insecurity is abnormal distress and anxiety in response to falling or the possibility of falling. *It is a primal fear.* It occurs when the child's brain overreacts to changes in gravity, even as subtle as standing up.

Movement for this child is not fun; it is scary. When her head moves, she responds, "I'm falling! I'm out of control!" She overreacts with a fight-or-flight response.

The fight response plays out as negative, defiant behavior, particularly when she is passively moved. She may resist being picked up, rocked, or pushed in the stroller. She may become angry and stubborn when someone suggests riding in the car or sledding down a hill.

How Gravitational Insecurity Affects a Child's Behavior

A Typical Child	A Child with SPD
With his class, Jack, nine, goes for a hike up a little mountain. At one point, a thick vine hangs down from a branch. Jack takes a turn swinging on the vine, screaming, "Tarzan!" Jack's efficient vestibular system permits him to enjoy exploring gravity as he swings and soars through the air.	The day his class goes hiking, Brad, nine, watches each step. He is grouchy, silent, and slow. He stands aloof while his classmates swing on a vine. When it is his turn, he takes the vine reluctantly. He cannot move. The others cry, "Come on! What's your problem? It's fun!" Brad senses that if his feet leave the ground, he will fall into the void. Saying "I am really not interested in this stupid game," he drops the vine and stalks away.

The flight response plays out as extreme caution or avoidance of movement. She prefers keeping her head up and feet down, firmly planted. She may avoid circle games, bicycles, slides, and swings. She may be fearful of unstable surfaces, such as a sandy beach or a climbing net at the playground. She may avoid novel experiences, such as visiting a friend's house, because any place other than home is unpredictable.

The child with this terror tends to be inflexible and controlling. She often has social and emotional problems, because she is so worried about falling that she always feels vulnerable when around other people. The result is that she cannot get organized for other tasks, such as playing and socializing.

Vestibular Underresponsivity—"Wait, What?"

A different child may be underresponsive to movement experiences. She does not respond negatively; she simply does not seem to notice. As an infant, she may have been "such an easy baby," always ready to curl up in anyone's arms, always ready for a long, long nap. As she matures, she seems to lack inner drive to move actively. Although she requires extra movement to "get in gear," this child does not usually seek movement. Once started, however, she may have difficulty stopping.

Also, the child may seem oblivious to a falling sensation. She cannot respond efficiently with protective extension, i.e., extending a hand or a foot to catch herself. Many children with autism with this difficulty may have bruises because of frequent falls.

How Vestibular Underresponsivity Affects a Child's Behavior

A Typical Child	A Child with SPD
Jeff, thirteen, comes to the pool for aquatic therapy to strengthen his leg, which he broke while skating. On the concrete pool deck, he slips on a puddle and reacts immediately to catch himself, reaching for the wall—so he does not fall and break the other leg!	Cameron, a thirteen-year-old with autism, comes to the pool for aquatic therapy. Lumbering toward his recreational therapist, he slips on a puddle. Unaware of the sensation of falling, and slow to protect himself, he ricochets off the wall and collapses on the pool deck. The therapist rushes to his side and guides him into the soothing water before he has a meltdown.

Vestibular Craving—"More!"

The child who craves vestibular sensations never seems to get enough of movements that are sufficiently satisfying for others. The sensory craver has an increased tolerance for movement. She seeks and enjoys a great deal of vigorous activity to satisfy her sensory needs.

To get vestibular sensations, the child may seek to resist gravity in unusual ways. For instance, she may assume upside-down positions, hang over the edge of her bed, or place her head down on the floor and pivot around it.

The child may frequently seek intense movement sensations, such as jumping from the top of the jungle gym or running fast when a sedate pace would do. Climbing may be her passion; for the sensory craver, everything is a ladder.

She may crave linear movement and enjoy rocking or swinging for exceptionally long times. She may especially seek rotary movement, such as twirling in circles, shaking her head vigorously from side to side, or spinning on a tire swing, merry-go-round, or amusement park ride.

She may flit and dart from one activity to another, always seeking a new thrill. Her attention span may be short, even for activities she enjoys. Although she may be constantly on the go, she may move without caution or good motor coordination.

How Sensory Craving Affects a Child's Behavior

A Typical Child	A Child with SPD
Justin, three, is at the swim center with his mother. He paddles in the kiddie pool, occasionally pausing to watch the big kids climb the ladder to the high diving board and jump into the water. When it is time to go home, he takes his mother's hand and says, "Let's go see that big ladder." He looks up longingly. It is so high! So scary! Someday he will be big and brave enough to climb it, but not yet.	Billy, three, is at the swim center with his mother. He starts to jump into the big pool, but she restrains him and guides him into the kiddie-pool enclosure. While she and the lifeguard discuss scheduling Billy's first swimming lesson, he escapes. He clambers up on the high diving board. He teeters on the edge, ready to jump into the deep water. His mother notices his absence, springs up the ladder, and catches him just before he falls.

VESTIBULAR DISCRIMINATION DIFFERENCES

"What Does That Mean?"

A child with superior vestibular discrimination may love to swing high and may aspire to become a flying trapeze artist. A child with vestibular discrimination difficulties, at the other end of the sensory processing continuum, is very different; her goal is to keep her head and body close to the ground.

How Vestibular Discrimination Affects a Child's Behavior

A Typical Child	A Child with SPD
Rachel, ten, enjoys games such as Pin the Tail on the Donkey at her birthday parties. She is comfortable being blindfolded and spun around, and she almost always sticks the tail close to the donkey's derriere.	Last year, Betty, ten, played Pin the Tail at Rachel's party and then threw up. She wants to participate in a different way this year. Her intelligent solution is to say, "I get dizzy doing this, so I'll help blindfold the kids and turn them around."

Head movements unsettle the sensory jumbler. Turning her head while sitting at her desk may cause her to fall from her seat. She may fall frequently while standing or walking. She may become easily confused when changing directions, going through obstacle courses, turning on her own axis, or circling in a folk dance. Bending over to pick a daisy, tie a shoe, or take a bow may throw her off balance. She may be unable to discriminate when just enough swinging becomes too much swinging, so she may keep swinging until she gets very dizzy or feels sick. When her eyes are closed or covered, she may be especially unsteady and resist moving, because vision helps her sense where she is in space.

How the Vestibular Sense Affects Everyday Skills

The vestibular sense gives us information necessary for many everyday skills:

- Gravitational security (see pages 142–43)
- Movement and balance
- Muscle tone
- Bilateral coordination
- Visual and auditory processing (see chapters 8 and 9)
- Praxis (motor planning)
- Emotional security

MOVEMENT AND BALANCE

Automatic, coordinated movement and balance are possible when the central nervous system connects vestibular sensations with other sensations. Movement and balance are sensory-based motor skills, not senses per se.

How Movement and Balance Affect a Child's Behavior

A Typical Child	A Child with SPD
When Jeremy, ten, first got his skateboard, he fell frequently, but he has gradually learned to adjust his weight to keep his balance. He sets up obstacle courses in the street, with ramps and traffic cones, and invites his pals to try new tricks. When Jim collides with him and throws him off balance, Jeremy can usually land on his feet.	Jim, ten, cannot get the hang of riding his skateboard, although he works hard every day to master this skill. Yet he still crashes into Jeremy's ramps and traffic cones, and even into Jeremy. Usually Jim feels himself falling but cannot stop himself. His postural background adjustments are ineffective and he keeps losing his balance.

The vestibular system tells us which way is up, and that up is where we want to be. When we are upright, we are alert and in control. To keep upright, we make subconscious physical adaptations, called postural background adjustments. These subtle adjustments allow us to stabilize our bodies, to correct and maintain our balance, and to move easily.

The child with vestibular differences moves too little or too much, with too much or too little caution. Her balance may be off, and her movements may be uncoordinated and awkward.

MUSCLE TONE

Muscle tone is the degree of tension normally present when our muscles are in a resting state. (Muscles never relax completely unless we are unconscious.) Muscle tone is a component of normal movement patterns. When we have good muscle tone, we usually take it for granted.

How Muscle Tone Affects a Child's Behavior

A Typical Child	A Child with Vestibular Differences
Kenny, four, pulls on his socks and his high-top sneakers. He does not yet know how to tie his shoes. He grips with his toes to keep the loose sneakers on his feet and thumps to his father for help. His father says, "You're growing so fast, soon you'll be able to tie your shoes all by yourself." Kenny says, "But I can make them twinkle. Want to see, Daddy?" He springs up, and when he lands, the heels of the sneakers light up.	Ted's father parks him on the bed and tries to push his limp feet into a pair of socks. "Can you help me, son?" he asks. "It seems as if I'm doing all the work here." Ted tries to cooperate, but his feet do not always do what he wants them to do. Finally, the socks are on. While his father wiggles Ted's feet into his sneakers, Ted sprawls backward on the bed. "Can you help me, please?" asks his father. "Too tired," says Ted.

If you lead a normal life and exercise sometimes, you probably have adequate tone when you are resting. If you exercise regularly, you probably have firm tone. If you are a couch potato, you probably have low tone, and—because the apple does not fall far from the tree—chances are that your child is a "potato chip."

The vestibular system, along with the proprioceptive system, strongly affects tone by regulating neurological information from the brain to the muscles, telling them exactly how much to contract, so that we can resist gravity to perform skilled tasks. Usually, our muscle tone is neither too tight nor too loose; it is just right, so we do not have to use much effort to move our bodies or keep ourselves upright.

The child with vestibular differences may have a "loose and floppy" body, or low tone. This is a postural problem that interferes with her movement. Nothing is wrong structurally with her muscles, but her brain is not sending out sufficient messages to give them oomph. Without that energizing oomph, the child's muscles lack the readiness or tension necessary to move with ease.

The sensory slumper may often lay her head on the table, or sprawl on the floor, or slouch in the chair. She may have difficulty turning knobs and pressing levers. She may handle objects loosely or with a very tight grasp in order to compensate for the underlying low muscle tone. She may tire easily, because resisting the pull of gravity requires a great deal of energy.

BILATERAL COORDINATION

An integrated vestibular system helps us use both body sides together as a team. Bilateral (from the Latin for "two sides") coordination is an important perceptual-motor skill—i.e., the child's ability to use his emerging sensory processing skills to learn about his environment by moving and interacting within it.

Components of bilateral coordination include:

- Symmetrical movements—jumping on a trampoline, catching a ball with both hands, playing clapping games, and pressing Legos together.
- Alternating, or reciprocal, movements—creeping on hands and knees, climbing stairs, pedaling a bicycle, and zipping a jacket.
- Dominant/nondominant hand movements—holding a paper while cutting or writing with the other hand, tying shoelaces, and threading a needle.

Bilateral coordination leads to lateralization, also called laterality. One side of the brain directs movement on the opposite side of the body, while the other body side is used for stabilization. Thus, either side of the body can move independently of the other. For example, a preschooler usually has established hand and foot preferences. She uses her nondominant hand to hold a bottle of bubbles and her dominant hand to dip a wand into it. She balances on one leg and kicks a ball with the other. An older child uses one hand to toss up a ping-pong ball and the other hand to whack it with a paddle.

Crossing the midline is another perceptual-motor skill emerging from bilateral coordination. This is the ability to use a hand, foot, or eye in the space of the opposite side of the body. As he grows, the child learns to cross his midline to scratch an elbow, sit with crossed legs, and read from left to right without moving his head.

What do challenges with bilateral coordination mean for the child with SPD? Difficulties may arise when using paired body parts together to jump and separately to zip. She may not have developed laterality, and so she may not have established a preferred hand for drawing. (Using either hand for drawing, painting, cutting, and eating does not mean the child is ambidextrous, that is, able to use both hands equally well. It means the child uses neither hand well, so she keeps switching to try to get the job done.)

Furthermore, crossing the midline may be challenging. It may be hard to track a bird in flight without breaking her gaze at her midline. At the easel, she may switch hands at midpoint to paint a horizon from left to right rather than use just one hand to sweep the brush across the paper. Learning to

How Bilateral Coordination Affects a Child's Behavior

A Typical Child	A Child with SPD
Chelsea, eight, is making a valentine. On a piece of red paper, she steadies a cardboard heart with her left hand and traces its outline with her right. She uses her right hand to cut out the heart and her left hand to hold and turn the paper. She makes four more valentines during art period.	Celia, eight, wants to make a pink valentine. She has difficulty steadying the cardboard heart on the paper while she traces. Her outline is misshapen but will have to do. She picks up the paper in her right hand and the scissors in her left. No, that is not correct; she switches hands. Instead of rotating the paper with her left hand, she moves her right hand, awkwardly holding the scissors, around the paper. Her valentine is not gorgeous, but she knows her mother will like it.

read words across the page is confusing, exhausting, and
unrewarding.

Four fun activities to develop and enhance bilateral coordination are on pages 278–79. Other books in the *Sync* series
suggest many more.

Poor bilateral coordination is often misinterpreted as a
learning disability such as dyslexia. In fact, this difficulty can
lead to learning or behavior problems, but it does not ordinarily
mean that a child is lacking in intelligence or academic ability.

VISUAL AND AUDITORY PROCESSING

The vestibular system is intimately involved with vision and
hearing. Please see the next chapters to learn more.

PRAXIS (MOTOR PLANNING)

Praxis, or motor planning, as you have seen, is the ability to
conceptualize, organize, and realize a complex sequence of unfamiliar movements. When our nervous system integrates vestibular sensations with tactile and proprioceptive sensations,
we have a good body scheme. When we have a good body
scheme, we can motor plan. When we motor plan, we can accomplish what we set out to do.

Adapting her behavior to learn a new skill may be very
hard for the child with vestibular challenges. For instance, this
sensory fumbler may be able to step into the bathtub, but she
may have trouble stepping into the car. She may have learned
how to roller skate, but may have difficulty ice-skating or roll-
erblading. If her CNS has not processed movement and balance sensations efficiently, then her brain cannot remember
how it feels to move in a certain way. Thus, she cannot easily

How Praxis Affects a Child's Behavior

A Typical Child	A Child with SPD
Maddy, seven, likes learning new dances. Today the Brownies are mastering the Macarena, a dance that their Brownie leader learned as a girl. In this dance, the girls move their arms and hands in a complicated sequence, turning them in the air and moving them to touch one body part after another. After completing the sequence, they shimmy, jump a quarter turn, and repeat the motions. The Macarena is much more challenging than the looby-loo. Maddy loves this.	Libby likes being a Brownie, especially going on field trips, but she dislikes dancing. The looby-loo was hard enough; now she must deal with the Macarena. Moving her arms and hands is confusing and frustrating. Shimmying is difficult, so Libby just sways. Trying to jump a quarter turn, she goes in the wrong direction. Learning the sequence of movements is so hard! She wishes they could stick to familiar activities instead of always tackling something new.

generalize a learned skill to plan and perform a new skill that is only slightly different.

How can you support a child with dyspraxia? OT-SI will help. At home and school, give the child plenty of time and space to practice challenging motor sequences. Offer objects with many "affordances" (see pages 271 and 278) for the child to explore using them in various ways. Whenever possible, go outdoors to dig in the dirt, walk through the woods, and play with nature.

EMOTIONAL SECURITY

Emotional security is every child's birthright, but the child with vestibular differences may feel insecure. With the inability to process where she stands and how she moves through space, she may be disorganized in many aspects of her young life.

The child may have a shaky sense of self and low self-esteem. Aware that ordinary tasks are beyond her ability, she may say, "I can't do that." She may not even try. If she is uncertain about her abilities, even the best-loved child in the world may feel unloved and unlovable.

How Emotional Security Affects a Child's Behavior

A Typical Child	A Child with SPD
Mark, four, gives Darius a huge, soft baseball and plastic bat for his birthday. After Darius unwraps the gift, Mark says, "Let's play!" A few children can wield the bat and whack the ball. Mark hits it over the fence. He claps his hands. "I knew I'd be good at this! Your turn, Darius." He offers the bat to his friend, but Darius frowns and turns away. When Mark's mother comes to pick him up, he says, "Darius didn't like the bat, Mommy, but that's okay. I had a good time at the party anyway."	Darius, four, opens Mark's present, but he does not want to play with the ball and bat. He knows he won't be any good. He watches the other children line up to swing the bat, but when Mark urges him to try, he turns away and says, "I can't." After the partygoers leave, he says to his mother, "Mark isn't my friend. He hates me." His eyes brim with tears, and he collapses in her arms. He whimpers, "Mommy, do you love me?"

Characteristics of Vestibular Differences

These checklists will help you gauge whether your child has vestibular differences that get in his or her way. As you check recognizable characteristics, you will begin to see emerging patterns that help to explain your child's out-of-sync behavior.

The sensory avoider with **intolerance for movement** may:

❑ Dislike swinging, spinning, and sliding activities.
❑ Be cautious, slow moving, and sedentary, hesitating to take risks.

❏ Appear to be very immature.

❏ Seem willful and uncooperative.

❏ Be very uncomfortable in elevators and on escalators, perhaps experiencing car or motion sickness.

❏ Demand continual physical support from a trusted adult.

The child with **gravitational insecurity** may:

❏ Have a great fear of falling, even where no real danger exists. This fear is experienced as primal terror.

❏ Be fearful of heights, even slightly raised surfaces. The child may avoid walking on a curb or jumping down from the bottom step.

❏ Become anxious when her feet leave the ground, feeling that even the smallest movement will throw her into outer space.

❏ Be fearful of climbing or descending stairs and hold tightly to the banister.

❏ Feel threatened when her head is inverted, upside down or tilted, as when having her head shampooed over the sink.

❏ Be fearful when someone moves her, as when a teacher slides her chair closer to the table.

❏ For self-protection, try to manipulate her environment and other people.

❏ Have poor proprioception and poor visual discrimination.

The sensory straggler with **underresponsivity** to vestibular sensations may:

❏ Not notice or object to being moved.

❏ Seem to lack inner drive to move actively.

❑ Once started, swing for a lengthy time without getting dizzy.

❑ Not notice sensation of falling and may not respond efficiently to protect himself by extending his hands or a foot.

The sensory-craver with **increased tolerance for movement** may:

❑ Need to keep moving, as much as possible, in order to function. The child may have trouble sitting still or staying in a seat.

❑ Repeatedly, vigorously shake her head, rock back and forth, and jump up and down.

❑ Crave intense movement experiences, such as bouncing on furniture, using a rocking chair, turning in a swivel chair, assuming upside-down positions, or placing her head on the floor and pivoting around it.

❑ Be a "thrill seeker," enjoying fast-moving or spinning playground equipment, or seeking the fast and "scary" rides at an amusement park.

❑ Not get dizzy, even after twirling or spinning rapidly for a lengthy amount of time.

❑ Enjoy swinging very high and/or for long periods of time.

❑ Like seesaws, teeter-totters, or trampolines more than other children.

The sensory slumper with **postural differences** affecting movement of the head, balance, muscle tone, and bilateral coordination may:

❑ Lose her balance unless both feet are firmly planted, as when stretching on tiptoes, jumping, or standing on both feet when her eyes are closed.

❑ Easily lose her balance when out of a biped (two-footed) position, as when climbing stairs, riding a bicycle, hopping, or standing on one foot.

❑ Move in an uncoordinated, awkward way.

❑ Be fidgety and clumsy.

❑ Have a loose and floppy body.

❑ Feel limp (like a wet noodle) when you lift her, move her limbs to help her get dressed, or try to help her balance on a teeter-totter or balance beam.

❑ Tend to slump or sprawl in a chair or over a table, prefer to lie down rather than sit upright, and constantly lean her head on a hand or arm.

❑ Find it hard to hold up her head, arms, and legs simultaneously when lying on her stomach.

❑ Sit on the floor with her legs in a W position, i.e., with her knees bent and her feet extended out to the sides, to stabilize her body.

❑ Have difficulty turning doorknobs or handles that require pressure, and have a loose grasp on "tools" such as pencils, scissors, or spoons.

❑ Have a tight, tense grasp on objects (to compensate for looseness).

❑ Have problems with digestion and elimination.

❑ Fatigue easily during physical activities or family outings.

❑ Be unable to catch herself from falling.

❑ Not have crawled or crept as a baby.

❑ Have poor body awareness.

❑ Have poor gross-motor skills and frequently stumble and trip, or be clumsy at sports and active games. She may seem to have "two left feet."

❑ Have poor fine-motor skills and difficulty using "tools" such as eating utensils, crayons, pencils, and combs.

❑ Have difficulty making both feet or both hands work together, such as when jumping up and down or throwing and catching a ball.

❑ Have difficulty using one foot or hand to assist the other during tasks such as standing on one foot to kick a ball or holding the paper steady when writing or cutting.

❑ Have trouble using both hands in a smooth, alternating manner, as when striking rhythm instruments together to keep a musical beat.

❑ Not have an established hand preference by the age of four or five. The child may use either hand for coloring and writing, or may switch the crayon or pencil from one hand to the other.

❑ Avoid crossing the midline. The child may switch the brush from hand to hand while painting a horizontal line, or may have trouble tapping a hand on her opposite shoulder in games like Simon Says.

❑ Have a hard time with organization and structured activities.

The sensory fumbler with **dyspraxia** (poor motor planning) may:

❏ Have difficulty conceptualizing, organizing, and carrying out a sequence of unfamiliar movements.
❏ Be unable to generalize what she has already learned in order to accomplish a new task.

The child who is **emotionally insecure** may:

❏ Get easily frustrated and give up quickly.
❏ Be reluctant to try new activities.
❏ Have a low tolerance for potentially stressful situations.
❏ Have low self-esteem.
❏ Be irritable in others' company and avoid or withdraw from people.
❏ Have difficulty making friends and relating to peers.

Vestibular differences may be your child's primary difficulty, while the tactile sense (chapter 5) and the proprioceptive sense (chapter 6) may be challenging, too. Visual and auditory processing are discussed in chapters 8 and 9.

7

How to Tell if Your Child Has SPD in the Proprioceptive Sense

One Nine-Year-Old at the Swimming Pool

Tony has tried to play team sports, but it is hard for him to get his body to work in a coordinated way. He hates it when other kids, including his siblings, say mean things like "You sure have a lousy sense of timing" or "Nobody picks you for a team because you don't help."

Knowing how Tony longs to participate in a sport, his mother persuades him to join the beginners' swim team at the neighborhood pool. After shopping for goggles, a team suit, and a new athletic bag, Tony begins to think that swimming might be okay. At least it does not involve hitting balls.

The first day of practice, Tony inches into the locker room. The other boys dart in and out, joking and laughing, while Tony struggles to change his clothes. He watches his every move carefully, especially when he ties the waistband string of his swimsuit. He wants to be sure that his suit is on right, so nobody will laugh at him.

He goes out to the concrete pool deck and heads for the coach. He walks awkwardly, thudding his heels. He is watching his feet, not where he is going. He collides with a chair, which clatters across the concrete.

The coach glances up and beckons. He calls, "Come on! Get your goggles on! Dive in! Let's go!"

Putting the goggles on is tricky because Tony cannot see what he is doing. By the time he adjusts them, the other kids have dived in and begun swimming toward the far end of the pool.

Tony does not know how to dive, so getting into the pool is another challenge. He goes to the ladder and faces the water. With his arms awkwardly stretched behind him as he clings to the railings, he tries to descend. Then he remembers to face the ladder, not the water. He turns around, gropes for the rungs with his feet, and backs slowly into the pool.

Tony begins to swim. He had swimming lessons, so he knows the basics. However, the pattern of his strokes is uneven. He stretches his right arm nicely but bends his left elbow too much, so he swims with a "limp." The result is that he keeps veering to the left and bumping into the rope.

Another problem is breathing. He concentrates hard— right arm, left arm, breathe, right, left, breathe—but he gets the sequence mixed up. When he breathes, his arms stop moving and he feels as if he is about to sink.

When he gets to the end of the pool, Tony is exhausted. The other kids are already swimming back to the other end. He is always the last one. He thinks maybe swimming is not such a good idea after all.

ATYPICAL PATTERN OF BEHAVIOR

Tony is out of sync with his body and moves in an atypical pattern. He strikes his heels on the pool deck to get additional information to his muscles and joints. His awkward gait makes him look like a robot.

Tony has poor body awareness. He cannot perceive how his individual body parts move or where they are in space. He relies on vision to figure out how to make his body move. Changing into his swimsuit takes a long time because he must watch his hands. Positioning his goggles over his eyes is hard because he cannot see what he is doing.

Another challenge is orienting his body to get into the pool. First, Tony has trouble aligning his body properly on the ladder. Then, when he remembers to turn toward the ladder and to back into the water, he labors to find secure footing on the rungs.

In the pool, Tony's swimming is irregular. His strokes are erratic because he has difficulty matching the movements of his two arms.

Tony works hard to swim; he likes the water and wants to be successful. He is easily frustrated, however, and decides that swimming is not his thing. Uncoordinated and unaware of his body, Tony has proprioceptive differences, and, as is common, dyspraxia and some vestibular challenges as well.

On the next pages you will find an explanation of how the proprioceptive sense is supposed to function, followed by an explanation of the types of SPD that sink Tony.

The Smoothly Functioning Proprioceptive Sense

Proprioception tells us about our own movement and body position. (*Proprio* means "one's own" in Latin and *ception* implies "reception of sensations.") Proprioception informs us:

- Where our body or body parts are in space,
- How our body parts relate to one another,
- How much and how quickly our muscles are stretching,
- How fast our body is moving through space,
- How our timing is, and
- How much force our muscles put forth.

This kind of information is fundamental for every move we make. Our reflexes, automatic responses, and planned action (praxis) depend on it. The self-awareness that proprioception grants lets us do our job, whether we are a master violinist, downhill skier, or salad chef . . . or an apprentice bicycle rider, cookie snitcher, or book-report writer.

Proprioception is both subconscious, such as when we automatically hold our bodies upright on a chair, and conscious, such as when we uncross our legs before arising from the chair. Sometimes teachers and therapists use the term "kinesthesia" to describe the conscious awareness of joint position we use in learning, and it means the same thing.

Proprioception is the "position sense" or the "muscle sense." Receptors are mostly in the muscles and skin, and also in the joints, ligaments, tendons, and connective tissue. The stimulus for these receptors is stretch. When muscles or skin stretch or contract, and body parts bend and straighten, messages inform the central nervous system about where and how the movement occurs.

We get the most and best proprioception when we actively stretch and tighten our muscles in resistive motions, against the pull of gravity—say, when we do a push-up or heavy work, such as hoisting a loaded laundry basket. When we are passively moved—say, when a salesclerk lifts our foot to insert it into a shoe—we get modest proprioception.

Even when we are motionless, we receive proprioceptive messages without being consciously aware of them. For instance, if you are seated right now and close your eyes, you are relying on proprioception, not vision, to tell you that you are resting in a chair. Are your feet on a stool? Do your hands hold this book? Proprioception gives you this information without the need to look at your feet and hands.

Muscle sensations that come through the proprioceptive system are closely connected to both the tactile and the vestibular systems. Proprioception helps integrate touch and movement sensations. Because they are so interrelated, professionals sometimes speak of "tactile-proprioceptive" or "vestibular-proprioceptive" processing.

Tactile-proprioceptive (or "somatosensory") discrimination refers to the simultaneous sensations of touch and of body position. This skill is necessary for such ordinary tasks as judging the weight of a glass of milk or holding a pencil efficiently in order to write.

Vestibular-proprioceptive discrimination refers to the simultaneous sensations of head and body position when the child actively moves. This is needed for throwing and catching a ball, or climbing stairs.

What do we need proprioception for? The functions of

proprioception are to increase body awareness and to govern motor control and motor planning. Proprioception contributes to visual discrimination; the more we move, the better we make sense of what we see. It helps us with body expression, the ability to sequence our motions and move our body parts efficiently and economically. It allows us to walk smoothly, to run quickly, to carry a suitcase, to sit, to stand, to stretch, and to lie down. It gives us emotional security, for when we can trust our bodies, we feel safe and secure.

Another very important function is to help modulate our arousal level. It brings us up when we are way down, and down when we are way up. Proprioceptive experiences calm and organize us, bringing us back to center when we have been under- or overstimulated in any of the other senses. For instance, the proprioceptive input from pushing against a wall, pulling on rubber tubing, or hanging from a trapeze bar can arouse a person who has been sitting all day. The very same input can calm a person who suffers from sensory overload in a busy classroom.

Furthermore, the calm and organization that proprioceptive input instills may last a couple of hours, and the person can tap into it to help himself function. Teachers, parents, and therapists who understand this phenomenon know that the best way to get children to settle down for a story or to do their homework is by first providing abundant opportunities for stretching and resistive activities.

An additional function of proprioception is the discrimination of movement in time and space. An example is tying shoelaces, which requires good proprioception of the muscles in the fingers coordinated with good visual and tactile discrimination. To know when to let go of one end of the shoelace, and how big to make a loop, and where to stick that loop, we need praxis, praxis, praxis. As an adult, you may be able to tie laces in the dark and in your sleep; imagine trying to do it without proprioception.

The Out-of-Sync Proprioceptive Sense

The inefficient processing of sensations perceived through the muscles and skin, as well as the joints and ligaments, causes proprioceptive difficulties. These are almost always accompanied by tactile and/or vestibular differences. Whereas it is common for a child to have only a tactile problem or only a vestibular problem, it is less likely for a child to have only a proprioceptive problem.

The child with poor proprioception has difficulty interpreting sensations about the position and movement of his body parts. His CNS is inefficient at modulating these ordinarily subconscious sensations. Whether underresponsive or sensory craving, he may be unable to use this information for adaptive behavior. He may show confusion when walking down the street, getting in and out of the bathtub, or putting on eyeglasses. He may tackle everything and everybody.

Discriminating where his body parts are and the rate and speed of his movements is difficult. Because he cannot monitor his gross-motor and fine-motor muscles, motor control and praxis are challenging. His clumsiness is frustrating. Other people perceive him to be a klutz.

When manipulating objects, he may exert too much or too little pressure, struggling to turn doorknobs and regularly breaking toys and pencil points. He may spill the milk every time. The child may have a poor grip on heavy objects, such as buckets of water, or on lightweight objects, such as forks and combs. He may also have difficulty lifting and holding on to objects of different weights.

Because of poor body awareness, the child needs to use his eyes to see what his body is doing. Ordinary tasks, such as orienting his body to get dressed, zipping a jacket, buttoning a shirt, or getting out of bed in the dark, become very difficult without the aid of vision. Unless the child can watch every move, he may be unable to match a movement of one side of his body with a similar movement on the other side.

The child may be fearful when moving in space because he lacks postural stability. Because each new movement and each new position throws him off guard, he is emotionally insecure.

The child with an inefficient proprioceptive system may have modulation, discrimination, and motor problems affecting his every move.

SENSORY MODULATION DIFFERENCES

Proprioceptive Overresponsivity—"Oh, No!"
The child who avoids stretching his muscles may be overresponsive to proprioceptive stimuli and probably has postural differences and sensory-based motor problems.

He may shun activities with a lot of sensory input, such as jumping, hopping, running, crawling, and rolling. He may resist getting into unusual positions, such as wriggling between the bars of a schoolyard climber or doing calisthenics in a physical education class. Not only active movement but also passive movement may cause high anxiety when he is tightly hugged or when someone moves his arms and legs. The child may be a picky eater or problem feeder because certain food textures require forceful, coordinated chewing that makes him uncomfortable.

How Overresponsivity Affects a Child's Behavior

A Typical Child	A Child with SPD
Nisha, thirteen, at a Japanese restaurant, tries squid for the first time. The texture is rubbery. As she chews, she compares the sensation to other foods she has had before. This is unlike other seafood, she decides, and more like licorice or gum.	At the Japanese restaurant, Tia, thirteen, wants to be a good sport, so she takes a tiny bite of squid. It feels like chewing rubber, which is not okay. She removes the morsel from her mouth and hides it in her napkin. Then she concentrates on the rice.

Proprioceptive Underresponsivity—"Wait, What?"

The child who is underresponsive to proprioception seems to lack the inner drive to move and play. He often has poor somatosensory (tactile-proprioceptive) discrimination as well as postural problems and dyspraxia. This child tends to "fix," e.g., jam his elbow to his ribs for more input when trying to write, to compensate for postural instability.

The child lacks "internal eyes" to help him "see" what his body parts are doing. He may have poor body awareness and be unusually clumsy with objects. The sensory straggler may not notice that he has been sitting for a long time in an uncomfortable position. The sensation of pins and needles may not bother him. He may have difficulty orienting his body to get dressed.

This child needs someone to act like an ignition switch to get him started. Parents and teachers may notice that he becomes more alert and organized after heavy work activity. A sensory-enriched life, including chores around the house and classroom, will help, as will sensory integration intervention that provides plenty of proprioceptive feedback to increase arousal level.

How Underresponsivity Affects a Child's Behavior

A Typical Child	A Child with SPD
Lily, twelve, has been sitting on the couch for an hour, engrossed in a Harry Potter book. She feels stiff and needs to move. She stands up, laces her hands together, and pushes them out in front, overhead, from side to side, and behind her head. She repeats the stretching sequence, this time with her palms facing outward. Ahh, her body feels much better. She is ready to help slice vegetables for dinner and set the table.	Dina, twelve, has been in one position all day, deep into Harry Potter. Her mother calls. Dina arises stiffly and stumbles to the kitchen to help fix dinner. As she tends to break dishes and cut herself while slicing vegetables, her mother gives her jobs that provide sensory input without doing any damage. Dina scrubs potatoes, mixes fishcake ingredients, squeezes lemons, and tosses the salad. Now she feels more alert.

Proprioceptive Craving—"More!"

The sensory craver is a "bumper and crasher." He craves active movement, pushing, pulling, making "crash landings" by throwing himself to the ground, and lunging into walls, tables, and people. He craves passive input to muscles and joints as well, such as strong bear hugs, and being pressed, squeezed, or pummeled while roughhousing.

Always seeking more proprioceptive input, the sensory craver may bite, kick, hit, and behave in a seemingly aggressive manner. Some sensory cravers will engage in self-stimulation, such as biting their own skin or banging their head against the crib or wall. These children benefit from sensory integration treatment with ample opportunities for vigorous proprioceptive input to decrease their high arousal.

How Proprioceptive Craving
Affects a Child's Behavior

A Typical Child	A Child with SPD
Before doing errands, Aaron, five, and his father go to the play-ground. Aaron likes to pump on the swing all by himself. Later, at the grocery store, he helps with the grocery cart. Pushing it forward and pulling it back feels good in his arms, abdomen, and back. On one thrust the cart accidentally bumps into the apple bin and a few apples go flying—one right into the cart! Aaron's father raises an eyebrow. Aaron restrains himself and just pushes and pulls the cart a little bit.	Erik, five, and his mother are at the grocery store. She is in a hurry and he is cranky. He refuses to ride in the kiddie seat, so she lets him push the cart. He repeatedly pushes and pulls the cart and then strikes his head on the handlebar. Head down, he cannot see where he is going and crashes into a barrel of peanuts. That felt good! Before his mother can stop him, Erik deliberately shoves the cart into a display of cantaloupes. Next time they do errands, Erik's mother will be sure that he has time to run and play beforehand.

PROPRIOCEPTIVE DISCRIMINATION DIFFERENCES

"What Does That Mean?"

A child with excellent proprioceptive discrimination easily adapts his muscle movements and body positions for self-help tasks, chores, and sports activities. A child with proprioceptive discrimination difficulties is different; he seems to be unfamiliar with his own body, as if he has not yet met his arms, hands, legs, and feet.

The sensory jumbler has difficulty positioning his limbs for putting on clothes, kicking balls, getting into and out of a car, or riding a bicycle. He moves his muscles in a jerky manner when bending and straightening body parts to march, touch his toes, or climb stairs. Adjusting his muscles for pushing, pulling, lifting, or carrying heavy objects like cartons and buckets challenges him. He has difficulty differentiating how much force to use to grip and manipulate pencils and small toys, sometimes dropping them and sometimes breaking them. While roughhousing or playing circle games, he often shoves, squeezes, yanks, and dive-bombs into his friends.

How Proprioceptive Discrimination Affects a Child's Behavior

A Typical Child	A Child with SPD
Omar is learning to tackle other boys safely in a middle-school football program. He figures out how to make the "just right" contact—not so roughly that he gets a penalty and not so lightly that the other player keeps his grip on the ball.	Playing football, Rasheed, twelve, rams into the other boys and often hurts them. He cannot seem to judge how much force to use. He often gets penalized for rough plays. His parents say, "He doesn't know his own strength."

Extra outdoor play, supervised roughhousing, and opportunities throughout the day to move and stretch help the child with poor proprioception. Provide opportunities for the child to push, pull, lift, and carry heavy loads. He needs these activities, and while he may complain at first, he will learn to like them!

How the Proprioceptive Sense Affects Everyday Skills

Proprioception works closely with the tactile and vestibular systems, so some functions overlap. These functions include:

- Body awareness
- Motor control

- Grading of movement
- Postural stability
- Praxis (motor planning)
- Emotional security

BODY AWARENESS

Efficient proprioception provides information about body awareness, an important perceptual-motor skill. The child with poor proprioception may be unaware of his body position and body parts.

How Body Awareness
Affects a Child's Behavior

A Typical Child	A Child with SPD
To settle the children down before reading a story, Jonah's preschool teacher leads a stretching exercise. She says, "Close your eyes and stretch one arm way up toward the ceiling. Bring it down and now stretch the other arm, way up high." Jonah, three, follows her directions without difficulty.	Mitch, three, keeps his eyes open during the stretching exercise. He looks at his right arm to make sure it is moving. When the teacher says to stretch the other arm, Mitch peeks at Jonah to see what he is doing. Attempting to imitate Jonah, he gets confused. He raises his right arm again rather than his left.

MOTOR CONTROL

Proprioception provides information necessary to coordinate basic gross-motor and fine-motor movements. The child with poor proprioception has difficulty controlling large-motor movements, such as getting from one position to another, and fine-motor movements, such as grasping objects.

How Motor Control
Affects a Child's Behavior

A Typical Child	A Child with SPD
Benjy, eleven, rounds up kids for a game of Horse. Each child chooses a spot, and everyone takes a turn to stand there and shoot the basketball into the hoop. With every missed basket, a player gets a letter—H, O, R, S, E. Benjy has good motor control and rarely accumulates all the letters to spell horse, which would put him out of the game.	Jasper, eleven, tries to play Horse on the basketball court. It is his turn and he takes the ball. His motor control is out of sync because discriminating sensations of body position and muscle movement is hard. He tries to catapult the ball into the hoop, but his muscles are too weak. He misses and gets an H. Then he gets an O, an R, an S, and an E. He's out.

GRADING OF MOVEMENT

Proprioception helps us grade our movements. Grading of movement means that we sense how much pressure to exert as we flex and extend our muscles. We can judge what the quantity and quality of muscle movement should be and how forcefully we should move. Thus, we can gauge the amount of effort necessary to pick up a fluffy dust ball, lift a heavy carton, or yank open a stubborn drawer.

Suppose you are at a picnic and you set down your lemonade on the table beside someone else's empty cup. Later, you return for another refreshing sip but pick up the other person's cup. You sense immediately that this cup is not yours, because it does not feel full. And how do you know? Proprioception tells you so!

Because the child with SPD does not receive efficient messages from his muscles and joints, he has difficulty grading his movements to adapt to changing demands.

How Grading of Movement
Affects a Child's Behavior

A Typical Child	A Child with SPD
Rosie, seven, is going to help paint the bike shed at camp. She carries a brush in one hand and a heavy paint bucket in the other. Walking to the shed, she adjusts her body to keep upright despite carrying different weights.	Ruth, seven, holds a brush tightly in one hand so she won't drop it. Her counselor gives her a bucket of paint. As Ruth cannot perceive how heavy it is, she cannot tighten her muscles to stand upright. She leans way over to one side as she lugs the bucket.

POSTURAL STABILITY

Proprioception gives us the subconscious awareness of our body that helps us stabilize ourselves when we sit, stand, and move. The child with SPD lacks the stability to make fundamental postural adjustments for these everyday skills.

How Postural Stability
Affects a Child's Behavior

A Typical Child	A Child with SPD
Larry, ten, pulls in his chair and surveys the dinner table. Yippee, corn on the cob! He eats with his elbows on the table. His mother says, "Manners, please," and he straightens up.	Adam, ten, perches on the chair: one foot tucked under his body and the other on the floor. His mother disapproves of elbows on the table, but he cannot help it when he eats corn.

PRAXIS (MOTOR PLANNING)

Praxis depends on accurate modulation and discrimination of proprioceptive messages. Planning and sequencing motor action is a challenge for people with dyspraxia, especially if they have underresponsivity.

How Praxis (Motor Planning) Affects a Child's Behavior

A Typical Child	A Child with Dyspraxia
Todd, six, is practicing a marching routine in preparation for Field Day. "Hup, two, three, four, hup, two, three, four," he chants as he smartly brings up his knees. When the PE teacher adds arm swings and counts faster, Todd enjoys the extra challenge.	Collin lingers at the end of the line as the first-graders practice marching. Even when he chants, "Hup, two, three, four," he cannot seem to coordinate his knees in a rhythmic pattern. Adding arm swings and moving faster make it harder. Collin shuffles along and mutters, "I can't do that."

EMOTIONAL SECURITY

Proprioception contributes to our emotional security by orienting us to where our various body parts are and what we are doing with our bodies. The child with SPD is not confident about his own body. Because he lacks the "feel" of it, he is emotionally insecure.

How Emotional Security Affects a Child's Behavior

A Typical Child	A Child with SPD
Jenny, five, gets out of bed, dresses, walks to school, does her worksheets, plays outside, and goes on errands with her mother. She feels good about herself and the world she inhabits. Her sense of security results, in part, from dependable messages coming from her body. She can easily orient her body, and this ability gives her confidence as she moves through her day.	For Sara, five, almost everything she does requires effort—getting out of bed, dressing, walking to school, doing her worksheets, playing at the playground, and going on errands with her mother. She does not feel good about herself or the world she inhabits. Her sense of insecurity results from the undependable messages coming from her body, which does not move the way she wants it to. She has little self-confidence.

Characteristics of Proprioceptive Differences

These checklists will help you gauge whether your child has proprioceptive difficulties. As you check recognizable characteristics, you will begin to see emerging patterns that explain your child's out-of-sync behavior.

The sensory avoider who is **overresponsive** to proprioceptive input may:

❏ Prefer not to move or be moved.
❏ Become upset when it is necessary to stretch or contract his muscles.
❏ Avoid activities such as jumping, hopping, running, crawling, and rolling.
❏ Be a picky eater or problem feeder.

The sensory straggler who is **underresponsive** may:

❏ Have low tone.
❏ "Fix" elbow to ribs when writing, fix knees tightly together when standing, or brace torso against desk to compensate for low muscle tone.
❏ Walk on tiptoes to get more proprioception in the feet.
❏ Break toys easily.

The sensory **craver** may:

❏ Deliberately "bump and crash" into objects in the environment, e.g., jump from high places, dive into a leaf pile, and tackle people.
❏ Stamp or slap his feet on the ground when walking.

❑ Kick his heels against the floor or chair.

❑ Bang a stick or other object on a wall or fence while walking.

❑ To modulate his arousal level, engage in self-stimulatory activities, such as head banging, nail biting, finger sucking, or knuckle cracking.

❑ Rub his hands repeatedly on tables.

❑ Like to be tightly swaddled in a blanket or tucked in tightly at bedtime.

❑ Prefer shoelaces, hoods, and belts to be tightly fastened.

❑ Chew constantly on objects, such as shirt collars and cuffs, hood strings, pencils, toys, and gum. The child may enjoy chewy foods.

❑ Appear to be aggressive.

The sensory jumbler and fumbler with **poor discrimination** and **dyspraxia** may:

❑ Have poor body awareness and motor control.

❑ Have difficulty planning and executing movement. Controlling and monitoring motor tasks such as adjusting a collar or putting on eyeglasses may be especially hard if the child cannot see what he is doing.

❑ Have difficulty positioning his body, as when someone is helping him into a coat, or when he is trying to dress or undress himself.

❑ Have difficulty knowing where his body is in relation to objects and people, frequently falling, tripping, and bumping into obstacles.

❑ Have difficulty going up and down stairs.

❑ Show fear when moving in space.

The child with inefficient **grading of movement** may:

❏ Flex and extend his muscles more or less than necessary for tasks such as inserting his arms into sleeves or climbing.
❏ Hold pencils and crayons too lightly to make a clear impression or so tightly that the points break.
❏ Produce messy written work, often with large erasure holes.
❏ Frequently break delicate objects, and seem like a "bull in a china shop."
❏ Break items that require simple manipulation, such as lamp switches, hair barrettes, and toys that require putting together and pulling apart.
❏ Pick up an object with more force than necessary, such as a glass of water, causing the object to fly through the air.
❏ Pick up an object with less force than necessary—and thus be unable to lift it. He may complain that objects such as boots or books are "too heavy."
❏ Have difficulty lifting or holding objects if they do not weigh the same. He may not understand concepts of "heavy" and "light."

The sensory slumper with **postural differences** may:

❏ Have poor posture.
❏ Lean his head on his hands when he works at a desk.
❏ Slump in a chair, over a table, or while seated on the floor.
❏ Sit on the edge of the chair and keep one foot on the floor for extra stability.

❑ Be unable to keep his balance while standing on one foot.

The child with **emotional insecurity** may:

❑ Avoid participation in ordinary movement experiences, because they make him feel uncomfortable or inadequate.
❑ Become rigid, sticking to the activities that he has mastered and resisting new physical challenges.
❑ Lack self-confidence, saying, "I can't do that," even before trying.
❑ Become timid in unfamiliar situations.

Proprioceptive differences usually coexist with tactile and/or vestibular differences.

8

How to Tell if Your Child Has SPD in the Visual Sense

Two Seventh-Graders at School

Few would guess that Francesca, twelve, has a visual problem. She is the best reader in the seventh grade and loves literature, such as *Oliver Twist*. All she ever does is read, read, read.

Today, after a quick lunch, she scurries from the cafeteria and heads for the library, her haven. She ducks to avoid other students darting through the busy corridor. She enters the library, locates a couple of titles about kites, and goes to an interior corner of the room. Sinking to the floor, she leans against a bookcase, faces the blank wall, and buries her nose in the books.

Francesca loves the tranquil library, where she does not squint or get headaches. The reason is that the library has full-spectrum light bulbs in the ceiling, unlike the flickering fluorescent lights in classrooms. Also, in her quiet corner, no sunlight glimmering through venetian blinds can irritate her sensitive eyes.

Along comes Charity, also with undetected visual challenges, looking for Francesca. Oblivious to most obstacles,

Charity bumps into a book cart. The cart tips over; books go flying. She clumsily gathers the books and shoves them back onto the cart.

Charity is often confused about where she is in space and has a poor sense of direction. Paying attention to words on the page or moving her eyes smoothly from one line to the next is also hard. Her strength is listening, so she does well in French and Spanish, poetry, and music. Charity is "smart as the dickens," as Francesca says, but not much of a reader.

Francesca hears Charity coming. "Hi!" she says, glancing up at her friend.

Charity has asked Francesca to scan the shelves for some titles, because that detailed visual job befuddles her. She whispers, "Did you find some good kite books? Any awesome designs?"

"Here's a butterfly pattern for you," Francesca says, "and here's the Baltimore oriole I want to copy." The girls admire the illustrations and whisper about the kites they will be crafting in art class. They are looking forward to an upcoming field trip to Washington, DC, to see the National Cherry Blossom Festival parade and to fly kites on the National Mall.

Later, in art class, they attempt to work on their kites and immediately run into problems. One problem is shifting their gaze from the book illustrations to their work and back again. Focusing and refocusing are hard. Another difficulty is transposing the designs they have chosen onto the kite wings. They cannot visualize how to enlarge the butterfly and the bird because relating the parts to the whole is a visual skill they have not yet developed.

The art teacher comes to their table and frowns at the girls' cockeyed efforts. She looks for something positive to say. "I see you are both working really hard."

The girls stare at her anxiously. Charity wonders if the teacher is angry. Searching her face, she is not sure.

"Hmm," the teacher says. "Next time, how about if you start over with something less complex? Sometimes less is more."

"Yes," agrees Charity. "Something simpler." She relaxes a bit. Maybe the teacher is not mad. At least, she does not sound mad.

Francesca sighs. "I guess I could just paint big dots instead of a bird."

The bell rings, and as the girls pack up to leave, the teacher gives them an understanding smile. She cannot understand, however, why such smart pupils struggle over an art project that ought to be well within their capabilities. Why can't Francesca and Charity make sense of images right before their eyes?

ATYPICAL PATTERNS OF BEHAVIOR

Why, indeed, can't Francesca and Charity make sense of what they see?

They both show atypical patterns of behavior. Francesca is overresponsive to visual sensations. Her body's way to compensate is with overaccommodation (a problem with a basic visual skill). Yes, she can read well, but most visual stimulation puts her on overload. She has difficulty negotiating her way through a busy hallway, tolerating flickering lights, and maintaining direct eye contact.

Charity's visual processing problem is different. She is underresponsive to visual stimuli. She has difficulty knowing what she is looking at, where it is in space, and where she is in relation to it. One problem is compression of visual attention;

she can focus on just one object at a time rather than see the whole picture. Compressed attention causes poor visual figure-ground (a discrimination problem). She cannot make sense of the cart in her path, the titles on the bookshelf, and the print on the page. She also misreads visual cues in facial expressions.

Additionally, both girls have visual dyspraxia. Their brains are inefficient at integrating visual input with motor output. Thus, their visual-motor responses are delayed and clumsy. They cannot easily use vision to guide their movements and carry out a plan, such as reproducing designs from the book illustrations.

On the next pages you will learn how the visual sense is supposed to function, followed by an explanation of the types of visual processing differences that dim these seventh-graders' view of the world.

The Smoothly Functioning Visual Sense

Vision is a complex sensory system that enables us to identify sights, anticipate what is "coming at us," and prepare for a response. We use vision, first, to detect contrast, edge, and movement so we can defend ourselves; and second, to guide and direct our movement so we can interact meaningfully in our environment, socialize, and learn.

The stimulus that triggers vision is light or a change in light. This stimulus is external, and we have no actual physical contact with it as we do with tactile, vestibular, and proprioceptive stimuli.

A unique feature of vision is providing both temporal (time) and spatial (space) information. We see things sequentially and, at the same time, we see a volume of space. For instance, when we read, we move our eyes from one group of words to the next. As we move our eyes to a new position, we see and take in another group of words. Vision lets us process an enormous volume of space in the wink of an eye.

That vision is so important to us now is astounding, because, in terms of evolution, vision is a newcomer to the nervous system. Smell was the dominant sense of our ancient ancestors and still is crucial for many animals. Today, vision is humankind's dominant sense for learning where we are and what is happening around us, or what may happen at any moment.

Vision should not be confused with eyesight, which is only one part of vision. Eyesight, the basic ability to see the big "E" on the wall chart, is a given. Eyesight is a prerequisite for vision. Either we see or we don't. We can neither learn nor be taught to see.

Interesting Facts about Vision

* 80 percent of the information we take in comes through the eyes.
* 80 percent of visual processing is responsible for what we see, and 20 percent is responsible for where and how we see.
* $66\frac{2}{3}$ percent of the activity of the brain is devoted to vision when the eyes are open. Three billion impulses come into the CNS every second; two billion of these are visual.
* 93 percent of human communication is nonverbal; 55 percent of communication comes from seeing the speaker's facial expressions and body gestures.
* 75–90 percent of classroom learning depends on vision.
* 90 percent of visual problems are never diagnosed.
* 25 percent of all school-age students have undiagnosed vision problems.
* 70 percent of juvenile delinquents have undiagnosed vision problems.

Vision, unlike sight, is not a skill we are born with but rather one we develop gradually as we integrate our senses. Growing up, we learn to make sense of what we see.

How? Through movement! Movement, the basis of all learning, teaches the eyes to make sense of sights, whereas sitting still to read or to gaze at the computer screen does not.

The vestibular and proprioceptive systems profoundly influence our vision. When we stretch and contract postural muscles to lie down, sit up, or stand on two feet, sensations bombard our brain and facilitate eye movements. When we move around, switch directions, and change the position of our body, head, and eyes, we strengthen visual skills. When we engage in purposeful activity, our eyes become better coordinated. Thus, movement, balance, muscle control, and postural responses are must-haves for proper vision development.

The tactile sense, too, has a huge effect on vision. The infant's hand grazes his toes, and he turns to see what he has touched. The preschooler handles an orange and pays visual attention to its tactile properties. Tomorrow he can see another orange and know that it is round, rough, solid, and just right for holding, squeezing, rolling, and tossing. The older student can visualize images, such as a pyramid, a police officer, or a pepperoni pizza without touching or seeing the real thing. To see well, countless concrete, tactile experiences really count!

The auditory sense affects vision as well. When we hear a sound, the auditory information reinforces our visual processing about its whereabouts. A door slams, a friend calls our name, or a bird warbles; we turn to locate and see the source of the sound. Also, hearing reinforces our visual processing about what is being said. For example, hearing or saying the word "apple" triggers a visual image of an apple.

Indeed, we need all our senses to develop vision, just as we

need vision to develop the other senses—including smell and
taste. The ability to know many sensory details about what we
see, such as a muffin's aroma and flavor, even before we eat it,
is the happy result of sensory integration.

TWO COMPONENTS: DEFENSIVE ("OKAY!" OR "UH-OH!") AND DISCRIMINATIVE ("AHA!")

Like the other senses, vision has two components. Our first response is always defensive (see chapter 4). Vision acts primarily
to protect us from danger. When light hits the eye, our immediate response is reflexive, i.e., involuntary and without conscious
control. Automatically, we make adaptive responses so we can
see clearly, for clear and single vision is an essential survival skill.

Basic visual skills—the unconscious mechanisms of
sight—include:

- Acuity, the ability to see the details of objects.
- Adjusting from dark to bright light, e.g., when we step
  from a dim hall into the sunlight.
- Accommodation in each eye so we can focus on objects
  at varying distances, both at far point and at near point,
  such as looking back and forth from the desk to a scene
  outside the window or copying math problems from the
  board into an assignment notebook.
- Detection of movement, such as the spider creeping up
  the wall, the car coming down the road, or classmates
  moving in the schoolroom.
- Binocularity (two-eyed vision), the ability to sweep the
  eyes together in a coordinated way and use them as a
  team to form a single mental picture from the images

that the eyes separately record, such as looking skyward with two eyes to see just one moon.

- Ocular-motor (eye-motor) skills, including steady attention on an object (fixation), efficient movement from point to point or word to word (saccades), and tracking of a moving object (smooth pursuits), such as a ball in the air.

With healthy working eyes as the foundation, we can get on with the discriminative component of vision, involving conscious higher-level cognitive functions. (Various terms are used for these functions, including "visual-spatial perception," "visual cognition," "spatial cognition," "form and space perception," and "visual discrimination," the term used here.)

Visual discrimination helps us refine details about what we see, where that object is in space, and how we stand in relation to it. This "what, where, and how" of vision guides our responses to what we see.

How Basic Visual Skills Affect a Child's Behavior

A Typical Child	A Child with SPD
Danny, thirteen, lives for baseball. He is a "physical genius," his coach says, in part because of his excellent visual skills. Up at bat, he easily keeps his eyes on the ball and shifts his focus quickly from a far point (outfielder Kerry) to a near point (home plate). When he pitches, good eye-teaming helps him see exactly where to place the ball. He is a "natural."	Until Kerry, an eighth-grader, got glasses and vision therapy, he was not a notable ballplayer. Now, up at bat, fixing his gaze on the pitcher and tracking fastballs is easier. When Kerry is in the outfield, he no longer strains to coordinate his eye movements. When he is very tired, he may still see double, but now he is one of the team's most valuable players.

Discriminative skills include:

- Peripheral vision—awareness of images that surround us through the sides of our eyes, primarily for detecting motion.
- Depth perception—seeing objects and spaces around oneself in three dimensions and judging relative distances between objects, or between oneself and objects, in order to descend the stairs and avoid stepping on cracks in the pavement.
- Stable visual field—discerning which objects move and which objects remain stationary.
- Spatial relationships—including directionality (judging how close objects are to other objects and to oneself) and laterality (with one's own two-sidedness as a reference, the awareness of right/left, front/back, and up/down).
- Visual discrimination—discerning likenesses and differences in size, shape, pattern, form, position, and color.
- Form constancy—recognition of a form, symbol, or shape even when its size, position, or texture changes, in order to match, separate, or categorize objects, or to know whether a letter is "u" or "n," "p" or "q," or "S" or "5."
- Visual figure-ground—differentiating objects in the foreground and background, to distinguish one word on a page or a face in a crowd.
- Visual attention—using the eyes, brain, and body together long enough to stay with an activity, such as reading, following directions, or looking at an object or person.

- Visual memory—recognizing, associating, storing, and retrieving visual details that one has seen previously.
- Sequential memory—perceiving words and pictures in order and remembering the sequence, important for reading and spelling.
- Visualization—forming and manipulating images of objects, people, or scenarios in one's mind's eye, a prerequisite for language development.
- Visual-sensory integration—combining vision with touch, movement, balance, posture, hearing, and other sensory messages.

With both components of vision in sync, first we see, and then we respond to what we have seen. Visual-motor skills are movements based on the discrimination of visual information. These skills gradually evolve and we learn to connect seeing with doing, or praxis. After much practice, we can coordinate the "what, where, and how" of vision with gross-motor and fine-motor movement. Is our sock covered with lint? We can pick it off. Is the pothole deep and wide? We can move around it.

Visual-motor skills include:

- Eye-hand coordination—the ability of the eyes to guide fine-motor tasks, such as manipulating toys, fitting round pegs into round holes, using tools, eating, dressing, writing, and following printed patterns to build block structures.
- Eye-foot coordination—the ability of the eyes to guide gross-motor activities such as playing hopscotch, stepping into the bathtub, and kicking a ball.

- Eye-ear coordination—the ability of the eyes to see a letter, integrate the message with stored auditory information, and tell a person how to say it or use it in a word.

The child who has developed visual discrimination and visual-motor skills has had much practice in looking around, moving around, and actively participating in a variety of sensory experiences. This child can recognize a hammer, an "R," and a trapezoid, whether it is right side up or upside down. In his schoolwork, he can line up columns of numbers and write neatly between the margins. He can sort through a jumbled drawer to find a matching pair of socks. He can categorize square, rectangle, and curved wooden blocks to construct a building.

On the move, he can read and follow a treasure map. He can judge accurately where objects are in space and steer clear of furniture and other obstacles. He can run toward the ball on a playing field. He can travel in the same direction as everyone else in a parade. He can ride a bike from garage to grocery store and home again.

An Example of Visual Skills at Work

Envision this scenario to understand how important all the components of vision are for survival: You are walking on the sidewalk beside a green park and notice a diagonal path cutting through to the opposite side. You veer off the sidewalk and take the path (directionality). You sweep your eyes (binocularity) from left to right (scanning) and sense that the park environment is peaceful. From the corner of your eye (peripheral vision), you espy a slight motion (detection of movement) coming from a big lump wrapped in a red blanket and lying on a bench (visual discrimination). You freeze so the lump will not notice you. From afar, you evaluate the scene. Could that lump be a person lying down (form constancy)? It looks like other lumps you have seen (visual memory). You focus so your vision won't be blurred (accommodation). You gaze at the lump, the bench, the tree, and the path (fixation) and concentrate on the whole scene (visual attention). Is this situation good, bad, or neutral? Where is the lump in relation to where you are and where are you relative to safety on the busy street (spatial relationships)? Can you find your way out of the park (wayfinding)? The lump stirs suddenly and you jump (visual defensiveness). Without hesitating to analyze whether to fight it, flee from it, feed on it, feed it, or mate with it, you make a self-protective adaptive response. You simply point your feet in the opposite direction and run (eye-foot coordination).

The Out-of-Sync Visual Sense

Dr. Ayres and her gifted followers have found that many children with learning disabilities have problematic visual differences. Usually, their brains are inefficient in coordinating visual discrimination and visual-motor skills with vestibular, proprioceptive, and postural mechanisms. In other words, their eyes and bodies are out of sync.

Erratic vision development is common in children with autism—although it is frequently overlooked. The child with autism often has poor eye contact and has difficulty attending to and giving meaning to objects and people in his environment. When he is visually stressed, he may squint and "self-stim" (flap his hands in front of his eyes). "Self-stimming" is a compensatory attempt to open up visual space, relax his compressed visual attention, and function better.

Of course, many children without autism have obvious or not-so-obvious visual difficulties, too. When these involve movement (tripping on air), posture (slumping at the desk), and body awareness (difficulty learning left and right), then chances are that the problem is sensory based and SPD is the root.

However, when difficulty involves visual discrimination without movement (such as matching colors or reading a map), SPD is not necessarily the root. The cause could be an acuity problem, such as nearsightedness, or an intellectual disability, such as Down syndrome. Determining the underlying cause of visual problems matters greatly so that the appropriate treatment will match the specific problem.

The child with SPD and poor vision may have one or more problems with modulating, discriminating, and using visual sensations to respond adaptively to the world.

SENSORY MODULATION DIFFERENCES

Visual Overresponsivity—"Oh, No!"
The child with visual overresponsivity responds dramatically to benign environmental stimuli such as contrasts, reflections, shiny surfaces, and bright lights. She may turn her eyes away from sudden, vivid, or flickering lights, perhaps shielding her

How Overresponsivity Affects a Child's Behavior

A Typical Child	A Child with SPD
Leah, eleven, is looking after her little brother at the playground. He toddles toward the swings. In the nick of time, Leah notices that he is in the direct path of a child swinging down in a wide arc. Without hesitation, she grabs her brother's arm and tugs him out of the way.	Dorothy, eleven, babysits for a neighbor. At the park, the toddler tugs Dorothy toward the swings. The rapid movement of the children on the swings alarms her. She closes her eyes to avoid the commotion. One of the swingers inadvertently knocks her and her little charge to the ground.

eyes with her hands, sunglasses, or a cap visor. The child may also be disturbed by moving objects, such as dangling mobiles or people bustling in a busy environment. She may duck when objects come toward her, such as a ball or another fast-moving child.

Visual Underresponsivity—"Wait, What?"
The underresponsive child may not pay attention to novel visual stimuli, such as holiday decorations or rearranged classroom furniture. She may not respond quickly and efficiently when objects come toward her—for example, when a beanbag is tossed her way.

How Underresponsivity Affects a Child's Behavior

A Typical Child	A Child with SPD
Connor, a fourth-grader, looks up at the homework assignment chalked on the blackboard. He copies the assignment in his notebook, glances up again to compare it to what he wrote to be sure he got it right, gathers his gear into his backpack, and heads for the door.	While other children copy the assignment from the board, Rex, nine, stares out the window. The teacher beckons him and says, "It may be easier to hear the assignment than to read it. I'll tell you what to write down." Rex is grateful but cannot hold her gaze. He stares right through her.

She may be unaware of bright light or sunlight. She may not blink or turn away from the dazzling light. She may stare at objects without seeming to see them or at people's faces as if they are not even there.

Sensory Craving—"More!"
The child who craves more visual stimulation than most children may clamor for excessive time in front of the television or

computer screen and may be attracted to bright, flickering lights, such as strobe lights or stripes of sunlight pouring through window blinds.

How Sensory Craving Affects a Child's Behavior

A Typical Child	A Child with SPD
The defective fluorescent light slightly annoys Lucy, four, but she ignores it during show-and-tell. Then it is time to play outdoors. After school, she goes to Lynne's. She joins Lynne briefly to watch a video until she gets bored and looks for some dress-ups to try on.	Lynne, four, gazes up at the flickering fluorescent light. The long "on" and brief "off" distract her from show-and-tell. After school, Lucy comes to her house to play. Lynne sits close to the TV and stares at a mesmerizing video, while Lucy slips away and tries on some dress-ups.

VISUAL DISCRIMINATION DIFFERENCES

"What Does That Mean?"

The typical child can distinguish specific qualities about what she sees. She can tell the difference between the people and things she looks at.

The child with poor visual discrimination sees—but does not perceive the meaning of what he sees. Instead of linking visual information with auditory, touch, and movement sensations, his brain may misconnect the messages. For instance, if connecting sights with sounds is a problem, he may not know where to look when he hears the teacher's voice. If connecting sights with touch sensations is a problem, he may not know— just by looking—that a nail is sharp and a hammer is heavy. If connecting sights with movement sensations is a problem, he may not swerve to avoid bumping into furniture. If all the sensory pieces don't come together in his brain into a unified whole, it is most challenging to adapt responsively to the sights his eyes record.

The child may be unable to match or separate colors, shapes, numbers, letters, and words. He may not distinguish words in print, even his own name. As he grows, he may stumble over similar symbols (▲/▼), letters ("q"/"p"), numbers (1,000/10,000), and words ("outage/outrage," "uninformed/uniformed," "Austria/Australia"). He may have difficulty focusing and concentrating on details in pictures, puzzles, Lego instructions, history books, geometric proofs, recipes, sewing patterns, and so forth.

How Visual Discrimination Affects a Child's Behavior

A Typical Child	A Child with Poor Visual Discrimination
Eden, five, studies a magazine page called "What's Wrong with This Picture?" She spots an upside-down 4 on a kitchen clock, a banana where a knife should be, and a spider in a line of ants marching toward a sugar bowl. Giggling, she tries to share the page with Opal, but Opal's inattention disappoints her.	Opal, a kindergartner with visual challenges, looks briefly at "What's Wrong with This Picture?" when Eden shows it to her. But Opal cannot easily pick out the visual details, so the page does not hold her attention. She shrugs and hands it back to Eden. She does not recognize Eden's disappointment.

The child may be unsuccessful at differentiating between objects in the foreground and in the background. He may not enjoy examining richly illustrated books such as *Where's Waldo?* He may misjudge which pieces fit into a jigsaw puzzle and be unable to spot a friend in a crowd.

He may misread important visual cues in social interactions, such as facial expressions and gestures, which make up more than half of our human communication. The inability to discriminate whether another person is scowling or smiling is a significant disadvantage!

VISUAL-MOTOR SKILLS

The typical child uses visual information to guide her planned and purposeful movement. With synchronized visual-motor skills, she can move her body efficiently, get from point A to point B, look at and copy a simple drawing or block structure, and see, reach for, and grasp an object.

The child with poor visual-motor skills has difficulty using her vision to guide her movements. Visual dyspraxia may cause problems in visualizing, planning, and carrying out a sequence of complex movements, such as rolling over in bed to see the alarm clock. She may overreach for objects. She may stumble up stairs. She may find it hard to walk on a balance beam, ride a bicycle, tie shoes, cut out paper dolls, spread butter on toast, or thread a needle. She may be bewildered, emotionally insecure, and "lost in space."

Poor eye-hand coordination may mean the child struggles to use his eyes and hands together. He may have difficulty manipulating toys and school materials, catching balls, using crayons and pencils, and fastening his clothes.

Poor eye-foot coordination will impede a child's smooth walking, running, and success on the playing field. Poor eye-ear coordination will interfere with his ability to see and then say a letter or word, and thus, with his speaking, reading, and writing skills.

How Eye-Hand Coordination Affects a Child's Behavior

A Typical Child	A Child with SPD
At snack time, David, three, pours juice into a cup, stopping just before the juice reaches the brim. After his snack, he works on a puzzle. One piece does not seem to fit. He studies it and realizes that it is upside down. He corrects his error and completes the puzzle. Then he does another, more complicated one.	At snack time, Freddy pours juice until the cup overflows. The teacher cleans him up and offers him a simple jigsaw puzzle. Freddy attempts to put in the four pieces but cannot get them to fit. Frustrated, he shoves the puzzle off the table. He asks just to sit in the cozy corner and hold the guinea pig.

The child with visual dyspraxia may be unable to plan ahead and solve problems in his mind's eye. He may look at materials, know something can be done with them, and be unable to recruit the visual functions and skills needed to make something desirable actually happen.

How Visual Praxis Affects a Child's Behavior

A Typical Child	A Child with Visual Dyspraxia
Howie and Curt, second-graders, are playing with toy soldiers. Howie's idea is to map out a battlefield in the sandbox, add pebbles and twigs, and arrange their armies in strategic positions. As the work progresses, he visualizes how to place his soldiers strategically—some behind a rock, others between leafy branches, and others behind sand hills. This is exciting and engrossing work.	Curt agrees that a battlefield in the sandbox is a good idea, but he has no design or strategy in mind. He has difficulty sequencing and using visual information well. He lets Howie propose and carry out his plan. Curt's side of the battleground is mostly open territory. He lines up his soldiers in parallel rows and waits for the battle to begin.

Poor bilateral integration and poor postural responses frequently interfere with visual-motor skills. The child may have difficulty coordinating both sides of the body and stabilizing his head, trunk, and limbs to function effectively and to support visual-motor skills.

How Postural Responses Affect a Child's Behavior

A Typical Child	A Child with SPD
At his table, Bennett, a first-grader, sits upright and reads the workbook instructions. He understands them, picks up his crayon, and connects the dots.	Clark, six, slumps at the table. He twists in the chair, trying to get comfortable so that he can read the workbook. He cocks his head this way and that. The words dance on the page.

Fortunately, help is available. A developmental optometrist can provide vision therapy to strengthen eye-motor control, visual discrimination, and eye-hand coordination (see chapter 10).

Also, when occupational therapists provide therapy using a sensory integration framework to alleviate vestibular, proprioceptive, and postural problems, vision often improves. If therapy is not an option, a sensory-enriched life with many visual experiences is essential to ensure adequate vision development. To move is to see!

Characteristics of Visual Differences

These checklists will help you gauge whether your child has visual dysfunction. As you check recognizable characteristics, you will begin to see emerging patterns that help to explain your child's out-of-sync behavior.

The child with a problem with **basic visual skills** may:

❏ Have headaches, eyestrain, or red, burning, itchy, or teary eyes.

❏ Rub eyes or blink, frown, and squint excessively.

❏ Complain about blurred images when looking at pictures, print, or faces.

❏ Complain of seeing double.

❏ Complain that words seem to move on the page.

❏ Turn or tilt her head as she reads across a page.

❏ Hold a book too closely, or lower her face too closely to the desk.

❏ Have difficulty seeing the storybook or chalkboard, and request to move nearer.

❏ Have difficulty shifting her gaze from one object to another, such as when looking from the blackboard to her own paper, and make errors in copying.

❏ Have difficulty focusing on stationary objects.

❏ Frequently lose her place on the page, reread words or lines, and omit numbers, letters, words, or lines when reading or writing, and need to use her finger to keep her place.

❏ Have difficulty tracking or following a moving object, such as a ping-pong ball, or following along a line of printed words.

❏ Fatigue easily during schoolwork and sports-related activities.

The child with **difficulty modulating visual sensations** may:

❏ Shield her eyes to screen out sights, close or cover one eye, or squint.

❏ Avoid bright lights and sunlight, perhaps preferring to wear sunglasses, even indoors.

❏ Be uncomfortable or overwhelmed by moving objects or people.

❏ Duck or try to avoid objects coming toward her, such as a ball or another child.

❏ Withdraw from classroom participation and avoid group-movement activities.

❏ Avoid direct eye contact.

❏ Experience headaches, nausea, or dizziness.

❏ Be unaware of light/dark contrasts, edges, and reflections.

❏ Be unaware of movement, often bumping into moving objects such as swings.

❏ Respond late to visual information, such as obstacles in her path.

❏ Seek bright lights, strobe lights, and direct sunlight.

❏ Seek visual stimulation, such as finger flicking, spinning, and peering at patterns and edges, such as ceiling and fence lines.

❏ Move excessively (squirm, fidget) during visual tasks, such as workbook activities.

The child with poor **visual discrimination** may:

❏ Have difficulty seeing objects in three dimensions (depth perception).

❑ Seem overwhelmed by moving objects or people because of a problem discriminating between what moves and what is motionless (stable visual field).

❑ Have difficulty judging relative distances between objects, such as letters, words, numbers, or drawings on a page, or between oneself and objects in the environment, often bumping into things (spatial relationships).

❑ Not understand concepts such as up/down, forward/back, before/after, and first/second. The child may have a problem stringing beads in order, following a pattern to build with blocks, or wayfinding (going from one place to another without getting lost, or finding one's way in a new place).

❑ Have difficulty in team sports that require awareness of position on the field or court and knowledge of teammates' positions and movements.

❑ Confuse likenesses and differences in pictures, words, symbols, and objects and have difficulty distinguishing properties of objects.

❑ Repeatedly confuse similar beginnings and endings of words ("tree/free," "fight/flight/fright," "table/tablet").

❑ Have difficulty with schoolwork involving the size of letters, the spacing of letters and words on the line, and the lining up of numbers (form constancy). The child may reverse letters ("b/d") or words ("saw/was") while reading and writing.

❑ Have difficulty differentiating objects in the foreground and background, necessary to distinguish one word on a page, or a face in a crowd (visual figure-ground).

❑ Be unable to form mental images of objects, people, or scenarios, to envision what she reads or hears, or to relate pictures and words to the "real thing" (visualization).

❑ Have difficulty describing thoughts and actions, both verbally and in writing.

❑ Be a poor speller.

❑ Have difficulty remembering what he did or saw during the day.

❑ Be unable to interpret how objects would feel just by looking at them; the child must touch the kitten to know it is soft and furry.

❑ Fail to comprehend what she is reading or quickly lose interest.

❑ Have a short attention span for reading or copying information from the board, and have a poor visual memory of what she read.

The child with poor **visual-motor skills** may:

❑ Have poor eye-hand coordination—the efficient teamwork of the eyes and hands necessary for playing with toys, using tools, dressing, writing, and academic tasks.

❑ Be unable to use her eyes to guide hand movements necessary for accurate orientation of drawings and words on a page. She may be unable to stay within the lines when she colors, and her writing may be crooked and poorly spaced.

❑ Have difficulty with fine-motor tasks involving spatial relationships, such as doing jigsaw puzzles, rearranging dollhouse furniture, and cutting along lines.

❑ Have poor eye-foot coordination and difficulty walking upstairs or kicking balls.

❑ Have poor gross-motor skills and difficulty moving on playground equipment, such as reaching for and climbing on monkey bars.

❑ Avoid sports and group activities in which movement is required.

❑ Have difficulty with rhythmic activities.

❑ Have poor coordination and balance.

❑ Have difficulty sounding out a word silently and then saying it, or may mispronounce similar words as she continues reading (eye-ear coordination).

❑ Orient drawings poorly on the page, or write uphill or downhill.

❑ Have exceedingly poor posture while at the table or desk, or may twist sideways or tilt her head in an unusual way to see the teacher or book.

❑ Withdraw from classroom participation.

❑ Have low self-esteem.

9

How to Tell if Your Child Has SPD in the Auditory Sense

A Third-Grader in Music Class

This is the first Monday after vacation, and May has a stomach-ache. She does not want to go to school because on Mondays the third-graders go to the all-purpose room for music. May hates the teacher, crabby old Miss Cross, who insists that the children sit still during the whole lesson. She is not attuned to children like May, who learn best by moving.

The children are practicing for the spring concert. When they come into the room, first they sit and sing folk songs. May mouths the words without voicing them because Miss Cross told her, "If you won't sing in tune, don't sing out loud." Miss Cross doesn't understand that May would sing in tune if she could, but she can't.

After singing, the children play instruments. Half the students play the tunes on their recorders, while the others ac-company them on drums, rhythm sticks, and other unpitched percussion instruments. Then the groups switch and repeat the repertoire.

May hates the recorder because she never knows if the note

she plays sounds as it should. She does not have good pitch, which is the highness or lowness of sounds in relation to one another. She may try to play B, for instance, but her recorder sometimes squawks out a tone that is too sharp and sounds higher, like C. The other kids sidle away, and Miss Cross glares.

Playing the unpitched instruments is somewhat easier, but May also has problems with rhythm, timing, and dynamics. She comes in late, cannot catch or keep the beat, and plays *fortissimo* when she should play *pianissimo*. May just does not "get it" when it comes to making music.

Today, the children enter the room and are surprised to see a new teacher. Mr. Harmon smiles as they sit down. He says, "I am your teacher now. Miss Cross decided not to come back after vacation. She gave me some tips about managing this class, but I am going to toss those tips out the window and do something different. Let's get our whole bodies into this music-making business. Everybody, up! Let's move!"

Instead of making the children sit, he has them stand in one spot and sing scales, bending to touch the floor and stretching toward the ceiling to match the ascending and descending notes. Then they move around the room singing songs. He instructs them to walk and sing slowly, run and sing fast, stomp and sing loudly, tiptoe and sing softly.

May watches the other children for a moment until she catches on. Once she gets moving, she loves the crouching, stretching, and locomotion. She is not merely hearing the music—she is incorporating it into her body. It is all beginning to make sense.

Finally, with their bodies and voices primed, the children pick up the instruments. With a new sense of pitch and rhythm in her body, May understands how she can transpose some of that feeling into the music. Playing the recorder is not so hard today.

Next Monday, May will be eager to go to school. Stomach-aches on music day? Unheard of!

ATYPICAL PATTERN OF BEHAVIOR

When processing sounds, May shows an atypical pattern of behavior. Her auditory processing problems are caused by a sensory discrimination difficulty.

She sings and plays the recorder out of tune because she cannot discriminate differences in pitch in the musical tones. She is off the beat when playing the percussion instruments because of her inadequate sense of timing and rhythm. She must look at the other children when following the teacher's direc-tions because hearing the instructions is not enough—she needs visual information to help her understand what she hears.

Many children with sensory discrimination differences also have modulation problems, but May does not. (She is not overresponsive to sounds; she is not unaware of sounds; and she does not crave loud and constant noise.) She is somewhat clumsy, but once she understands Mr. Harmon's expectations, her body movements and motor planning improve.

The Smoothly Functioning Auditory Sense

The vestibular and auditory systems work together as they pro-cess sensations of movement and sound. These sensations are closely intertwined, because they both begin to be processed by special hair cells in the receptors of the ear.

Hearing, or audition, is the ability to receive sounds. We are born with this basic skill. We cannot learn how to do it; either we hear or we don't.

Auditory skills begin developing in the womb. The auditory nervous system is the first to become functional. In tandem with the vestibular system, it connects with muscles throughout the body and helps to regulate movement, equilibrium, and coordination.

The ear's influence on physical development is profound. Indeed, the ear is vital not only for hearing, balance, and flexibility but also for bilateral coordination, respiration (breathing), speaking, self-esteem, social relationships, vision, and, of course, academic learning.

TWO COMPONENTS: DEFENSIVE ("OKAY!" OR "UH-OH!") AND DISCRIMINATIVE ("AHA!")

The auditory sense, like the other senses, begins with a defensive component. As babies, we startle when we hear loud or unexpected noise. Gradually, our brains develop the ability to modulate sensations and tell us whether the sound is one we can enjoy and use or one we must avoid for self-protection. When we realize that a sound was just a door shutting and not a danger, we return to a state of being calm and alert.

The abilities to hear and to modulate sensations of sound underlie our ability to really listen to sounds around us and understand their meaning. We are not born with the skill of listening; we acquire it as we integrate vestibular and auditory sensations. Gradually, as we interact purposefully with our environment, we learn to interpret what we hear and to develop sophisticated auditory discrimination skills.

The discriminative component of the auditory sense evolves as the child moves, touches, and engages in many multisensory experiences. Discriminative functions, which help us refine details about the "what" and "where" of sounds, include:

- Localization—the ability to identify the source of a sound, such as a parent's voice or a friend's "Yoo-hoo!," and to judge the distance between the sound and oneself.

- Tracking—the ability to follow a sound, such as a helicopter as it putters across the sky or someone's footsteps as he patters around the house.

- Auditory memory—the ability to remember what was heard, e.g., conversations, directions, homework assignments, or song lyrics, and to refer to it at once (immediate memory) or later (deferred memory).

- Auditory sequencing—the ability to put in order what was heard and repeat it in logical order, such as the alphabet, Spanish verb conjugations, or multisyllabic words like "obstacle" or "nuclear."

- Auditory discrimination—the ability to compare and contrast environmental sounds, such as a food blender and a vacuum cleaner, and to hear likenesses and differences in word sounds, such as "road/load," "flute/fruit," "cup/cut."

- Auditory figure-ground—the ability to distinguish between foreground and background sounds in order to hear the main message without being distracted.

- Association—the ability to relate a novel sound to a familiar sound, such as connecting the bark of the neighbor's new puppy to the category of "dog," and the ability to relate a visual symbol, such as an alphabet letter or a musical note, with its particular sound.

- Auditory cohesion—the higher-level listening ability to unite various ideas into a coherent whole; to draw inferences from what is said; to understand riddles, jokes, puns, and verbal math problems; and to take notes in class.

- Auditory attention—the ability to maintain focus sufficiently to listen to a teacher's lesson, a conversation, or a story, essential for bringing the other auditory processing skills together.

An Example of Auditory Skills at Work

You attend Field Day at your child's school. Two hundred adults and children are milling about, talking, and laughing. All around, the decibel level is high, but you get used to it. Unexpectedly, a physical education teacher right behind you yells instructions through a bullhorn. You duck and cover your ears. What was he shouting? You are not sure because you had to shut out the noise. He moves down the sidelines. Aha, now you can listen to his message about lining up by classes (auditory attention). You hear a different sound now—it is a drummer (auditory discrimination) leading the band from the school building toward the crowd (tracking). You find yourself marching to the steady beat (ear-body coordination) as you move along the edge of the field. You look for your child but do not see her. Through the din, you hear her calling, "Hi, Mom!" (figure-ground). You turn to the source of the sound (localization) and wave to your child across the field. Then the band strikes up the national anthem. The crowd hushes. Everyone sings (auditory memory). Another parent says, "Isn't this great?" You nod (receptive language) and reply, "Field Day is always fun!" (expressive language). The games begin.

When defensive and discriminative components are in sync, we can respond adaptively to sounds. We know what the sounds are and where they come from, or can make educated guesses based on previous sounds we have heard. With information about the "what" and "where" of sounds, we develop auditory-motor coordination—what I call "ear-body coordination"—and learn how and when to move in accordance with the sounds. Our infant's hungry cry makes us prepare to nurse. A harsh tirade makes us cringe, rush-hour honking makes us tense, and clear, orderly music, such as Mozart's, makes us alert and organized.

When we process sounds typically, we can put out the uniquely human products of speech and language. Speech and language are entwined but not the same. Speech is the physical production of sound. Speech depends on smoothly functioning muscles in the throat, tongue, lips, and jaw. The vestibular, proprioceptive, and tactile systems govern motor control and motor planning for using those fine muscles to produce intelligible speech.

Language is the means to communicate with other human beings. It is a code for deciphering the meaning of words, which are symbols representing concrete objects and abstract ideas. Language is also the meaningful use of nonverbal gestures and facial expressions.

As we grow, we integrate what we hear with what we see and develop "social pragmatics." Social pragmatics are language skills we need to relate to others. We learn to understand what the other person is communicating, how the other person may be feeling, why it is important to show interest in the other person's ideas and conversation, when it is our turn to talk (or not talk), and so forth.

Language that we take in and understand, through listening and reading, is called "receptive." Receptive language focuses on external sounds, i.e., voices of other people and the noises all around us.

Language that we put out to communicate, through speaking, singing, or writing, is "expressive." Expressive language focuses on sounds we hear internally and that we reproduce, as accurately as possible, through our own voice.

We listen, move, speak, and read with our ear. Body awareness, balance, motor coordination, muscle control, postural responses, sequencing, language skills, planning ahead, and problem-solving grow stronger as we process the sounds that surround us.

The Out-of-Sync Auditory Sense

An auditory processing problem often occurs along with SPD. However, this problem can also stand alone, as the result, perhaps, of ear infections or hearing loss.

With or without SPD, a child may hear adequately but process sounds slowly or inaccurately. She may have a problem modulating or discriminating sensations of sound. Or she may be dyspraxic and come to a standstill when she hears sounds, not knowing how or when to start or stop an activity. Her rhythm and timing is off, affecting how she moves, reads, and communicates.

Her language may suffer. Recalling what she wants to say, putting her thoughts in order, or getting the words out may be hard. She may have a problem pronouncing words clearly enough to be understood. She may lack awareness of how her mouth, lips, and tongue feel and work together. She may say "tool" instead of "school," or "dese" instead of "these," because of difficulty positioning the muscles necessary for articulation.

SENSORY MODULATION DIFFERENCES

Auditory Overresponsivity—"Oh, No!"

For most of us, most of the time, when loud noises come at us, a muscle in the middle ear contracts to stifle the vibrations. This mechanism protects us from being overwhelmed or deafened. However, when we feel threatened ("Uh-oh!") and go into fight/flight/freeze mode, this little muscle does not clamp down. Instantly, keen attention to all sounds is imperative.

People whose auditory defensiveness keeps them constantly alert must listen to every sound. Easily distracted, some respond to ordinary noise with an infantile, whole-body startle. This state of ceaseless, on-edge alertness uses up energy, interferes with learning, and hampers language development and social interactions.

People with autism (and others, too, of course) often have auditory overresponsivity, or auditory defensiveness. Sounds that please others, such as chirping birds or rustling leaves, can make them feel as if their eardrums are being scraped.

With or without autism, the sensory avoider reacts strongly, swiftly, and negatively to loud, unexpected noises. He will alert to most sounds—even sounds that are too faint or high-pitched for most people to hear. When he hears sirens blaring, block towers tumbling, or people chewing, he may complain or cover his ears. Indeed, this child may worry incessantly about the possibility of loud noises, and that worry may affect his behavior.

If the metallic twang of guitar strings hurts, he may hang back from sing-alongs. If the sound of a balloon popping distresses him, he may refuse to go to birthday parties. If the rock concert promises a big sound, he may prefer an evening home alone. If he cannot get away from the hubbub, he may raise his

How Overresponsivity Affects a Child's Behavior

A Typical Child	A Child with SPD
Before lunch, Brynna, a fifth-grader, rushes to the school bathroom. The flushing toilets and whirring hand dryers are loud, but these everyday sounds do not bother her. When she hears loud, sudden noises such as screeching tires or fire alarms, she pays attention and winces. Otherwise, she briefly perks up her ears to unexpected sounds, such as books falling off a desk, and then ignores them.	When Nelia, ten, gets home from school, she rushes to the bathroom. She never goes at school because the noise of the toilet hurts her ears. The flushing water is as deafening as Niagara Falls. Nelia also jumps out of her skin and claps her hands over her ears when a pencil hits the floor or a door clicks shut. Her oversensitivity to sounds makes everyone refer to her as "Nervous Nellie."

own voice, hollering, "La-la-la-la!" to counteract the noise, rather like fighting fire with fire.

Auditory Underresponsivity—"Wait, What?"
The sensory straggler seems unaware of sounds that others hear and listen to. But is the child who seems unaware truly

How Underresponsivity Affects a Child's Behavior

A Typical Child	A Child with SPD
At the playground, kindergartners Asher and Frankie are playing with trucks at the base of the monkey bars. Another little boy, Jed, is climbing overhead and prepares to let go. He says, "Look out, look out!" Asher leaps nimbly out of the way, just in the nick of time.	Frankie is crouching under the monkey bars, engrossed with his truck. He hears Jed cry, "Look out!"—but does not respond and continues his play. Jed lets go and lands nearby. Startled, Frankie whimpers, "Don't do that." Jed says, "I told you I was gonna jump, you baby."

unaware? In many cases, we do not know. Children with autism, for example, who cannot clearly express themselves, may sense more than we can detect merely by looking at them.

The child with underresponsivity to sound does not visibly respond to quiet sounds, soft voices, and whispers that may be "under his radar." Likewise, he does not seem to respond to ordinary sounds, voices, questions, and comments. And when he does respond, he may speak very softly, almost in a whisper.

Sensory Craving—"More!"

The sensory craver loves crowds and places with noisy action like rodeos, car races, and parades. He welcomes loud noises and usually wants to turn the volume up. He may make his own noisy sounds, using his "outside voice" in the classroom and kitchen, and clapping and singing boisterously.

How Sensory Craving Affects a Child's Behavior

A Typical Child	A Child with SPD
Gwen, seven, is playing at Kaneesha's. Gwen covers her ears when her friend makes the TV louder. "Ouch! Let's do something else," Gwen says. The girls decide to make spoon bells. They each take a yard-long string, tie a large spoon in the middle, wrap the string ends around their index fingers, and bring them to their ears. They lean forward and tap the dangling spoons on the kitchen counter, tables, and chairs. A gentle tap sends vibrations up the string to Gwen's ears. Gong! Just like a church bell!	Kaneesha and her friend Gwen cannot agree about the TV volume. Gwen likes it low, and Kaneesha likes it so loud that she can feel the vibrations through her chair. Instead of arguing, the girls make spoon bells and walk around the kitchen, banging their spoons against the counters and furniture. Kaneesha pulls out an oven rack and hits her spoon on it forcefully to get a big bang. Wow! She scrapes the spoon across the crossbars. She loves the metallic reverberations. The racket is music to her ears.

AUDITORY DISCRIMINATION DIFFERENCES

"What Does That Mean?"

The child with SPD may have difficulty detecting likenesses and differences in words. She may find it hard to pick out or attend to the teacher's voice without being distracted by background noises. Her receptive language may suffer: She may be a poor listener and struggle to read. She may seem noncompliant or may not follow directions well, because she cannot decode what was said. Her expressive language may be inadequate: She may have difficulty participating in conversations, answering questions, and putting her thoughts into writing.

These differences from the way most children understand sounds may be obvious or, sadly, they may be entirely overlooked. Although the sensory jumbler strives to hear and listen, adults and other children may think he is willfully "just not paying attention!"

How Auditory Discrimination Affects a Child's Behavior

A Typical Child	A Child with SPD
Daisy's preschool teacher sings, "This old man, he played two, he played knick-knack on my . . ." She pauses and invites her four-year-old students to fill in the rhyme. Someone says, "Shoe!" Daisy says, "No, not shoe this time. Goo!" The teacher and most of the children laugh. "Goo" rhymes with "two," so it meets the criterion, and it certainly is silly!	"This old man, he played four, he played knick-knack on my . . ." The teacher leans toward Joni and invites her to supply a rhyming word. "Five!" Joni says. "Tell me a word that sounds like 'four,'" the teacher says. "Six!" Joni says. Her difficulty with auditory discrimination and cohesion means she neither understands the task nor the joke.

A phenomenon often observed is that a child who ordinarily does not talk much or well will begin to speak once she gets moving. Indeed, when she runs or swings, or bounces on a therapy ball, she may suddenly shout, sing, or talk. As self-therapy, to start verbalizing her thoughts, she may jump up to walk around the room. Active movement primes the pump, and speech begins to flow.

The child with movement and language challenges benefits greatly from therapy that simultaneously addresses both difficulties, because the vestibular and auditory systems are closely connected. Speech-and-language therapists report that putting the child in a swing during treatment can have remarkable results. Occupational therapists find that when treating a child for vestibular problems, speech-and-language skills improve along with balance, movement, and motor planning. Other treatments include auditory training based on the method developed by Alfred Tomatis, which improves the rhythm of movement and of language. (See page 260.)

Some improvements that children experience with auditory training include:

- Attention span and focus
- Social interactions
- Speech and motor control
- Auditory discrimination and sensitivity
- Musical expression
- Self-esteem, mood, and motivation
- Understanding spoken language
- Reading, spelling, and handwriting
- Bilateral coordination
- Physical balance and posture

Other ways to help the schoolchild with auditory difficulties include softening the sound in a noisy classroom, perhaps with a carpet; placing the child in a spot as far from bubbling fish tanks and doorways as possible; and using visual cues to help him supplement the auditory information he may miss.

Determining the cause of a child's hearing difficulties is important in order to treat it appropriately. When SPD is the root, a speech/language pathologist or an occupational therapist trained to provide sensory integration therapy is the logical choice. When SPD is not the cause of hearing problems, professionals who provide advice and treatment might include a pediatrician, an otologist (a medical doctor specializing in ear diseases), or an audiologist (a specialist in evaluating hearing disabilities).

How Movement Affects a Child's Auditory Function

A Typical Child	A Child with SPD
The fourth-graders cannot go outside for recess because it is raining, so Hayley chats with her friends as they work on a jigsaw puzzle. When math begins after recess, the kids cannot settle down. The teacher begins the class with the "Hokey Pokey." Shaking her arms, legs, and head and turning herself about, Hayley begins to feel alert again. When the teacher asks her for the answer to a math problem, Hayley responds correctly.	Caitlin misses recess on rainy days. Restless, she wanders around the room. The "Hokey Pokey" does not help, as she cannot understand the directions. She feels sleepy when math begins. The teacher asks her an easy question. She can't answer. The next day is sunny, and the kids go out. Caitlin swings the whole time. Later, the teacher asks another math question. Caitlin gets it right. The teacher wonders why Caitlin is sometimes "on" and sometimes "off."

Characteristics of Auditory Differences

These checklists will help you gauge whether your child has auditory differences. As you check recognizable characteristics, you will begin to see emerging patterns that help to explain your child's out-of-sync behavior.

The child with **difficulty modulating auditory sensations** may:

❑ Be distressed by loud noises, including the sound of voices.

❑ Be distressed by sudden noises, such as thunder, fire alarms, sirens, and balloons popping.

❑ Be distressed by tinny or metallic sounds, such as those coming from a xylophone or from clinking silverware.

❑ Be distressed by high-pitched sounds, such as those coming from whistles, violins, sopranos, and screeching chalk.

❑ Be distressed by sounds that do not bother others, such as a toilet flushing, a distant church bell, or soft music.

❑ Seek sounds that would be loud or annoying to others.

With poor **auditory discrimination**, the child may:

❑ Seem unaware of the source of sounds or may look all around to locate where they come from.

❑ Have difficulty recognizing particular sounds, such as voices or cars coming down the street.

❑ Have difficulty tracking a sound in the environment, such as footsteps.

❑ Have difficulty recalling, repeating, and referring to words, phrases, conversations, song lyrics, or instructions, both right away (immediate memory) and later (deferred memory).

❑ Have difficulty recognizing the difference between sounds, such as near or distant banging, angry or pleasant voices, or high or low notes.

❑ Be unable to maintain attention to a voice, conversation, story, or sound without being distracted by other sounds.

❑ Have difficulty associating new sounds to familiar sounds, or visual symbols (letters, numerals, musical notes) to their particular sounds.

❑ Have difficulty hearing or reading jokes, verbal math problems, crossword puzzle definitions, or discussions, and understanding how all the information fits together into a coherent whole.

❑ Have a poor sense of timing and rhythm when clapping, marching, singing, jumping rope, or playing rhythm band instruments.

The child may also have difficulty with **receptive language** and may:

❑ Have a problem discriminating between similar word sounds, especially consonants at ends of words, as in "cap/cat," "bad/bag," "side/sign."

❑ Have a short attention span for listening to stories or for reading.

❑ Misinterpret questions and requests.

❑ Be able to follow only one or two instructions in sequence.

❑ Look to others before responding.
❑ Frequently ask for repetition, or be less likely than others to ask for clarification of ambiguous directions or descriptions.
❑ Have difficulty recognizing rhymes.
❑ Have difficulty learning new languages.

The child may have difficulty with **expressive language** and may:

❑ Have been a late talker.
❑ Have difficulty putting thoughts into spoken or written words.
❑ Talk "off topic," e.g., talk about her new shirt when others are discussing zoo animals or a soccer game.
❑ Have difficulty "closing circles of communication," i.e., responding to others' questions and comments on demand.
❑ Have difficulty correcting or revising what she has said so that others can understand.
❑ Have a weak vocabulary.
❑ Use immature sentence structure (poor grammar and syntax).
❑ Have poor spelling skills.
❑ Have a limited imagination in fantasy play.
❑ Have difficulty making up rhymes.
❑ Sing out of tune.
❑ Have difficulty with reading, especially out loud.
❑ Require more time than other children responding to sounds and voices.

The child may have difficulty with **speech and articulation**, and may:

❑ Be unable to speak clearly enough to be understood.
❑ Have a flat, monotonous voice quality.
❑ Speak very loudly or very softly.
❑ Speak with a hoarse, husky, strident, weak, or breathy voice.
❑ Speak hesitantly or without fluency and rhythm.

In general, the child may:

❑ Be tired at the end of the day.
❑ Have little motivation or interest in schoolwork.
❑ Have difficulty planning tasks and getting organized.
❑ Be awkward and uncoordinated in movement.
❑ Have poor timing and poor athletic skills.
❑ Have low self-esteem.
❑ Be shy and tend to withdraw from social scenes.
❑ Improve the ability to speak while or after experiencing intense movement.

Part 2 of this book will give you specific, practical advice as you begin the process of evaluation, diagnosis, and treatment. You will also find many suggestions and activities to help your child at home and at school.

Coping with Sensory Processing Differences

10

Diagnosis and Treatment

This chapter will help you learn to recognize and document your child's out-of-sync behavior. It suggests when and how to seek a professional evaluation and diagnosis. It includes descriptions of various kinds of intervention, with emphasis on OT-SI, which is occupational therapy (OT) using a sensory integration (SI) framework.

A Parent's Search for Answers

A mother wrote me this letter:

> By the time Rob was two, I felt he had a special need, but I couldn't figure out what it was. He required constant attention. Time-outs didn't work because I couldn't contain him. He was defiant, disobedient, disrespectful, and demanding. He was always busy, always talking (great verbal skills!), strong-willed, contrary, and easily frustrated. I felt blessed to have Rob, and wouldn't trade him for the world, of course, but he constantly tested and rejected me.
>
> What was the reason for his behavior? How could I regain control? What method of discipline would get through to him? If

his behavior was an attempt to get my attention, how could I supply it in a way that would satisfy him? How could I help a high-energy child channel his energy in a positive direction? I was desperate for answers.

I started seeking information from my pediatrician. He recommended a neurologist, who tested Rob for seizures (he tested normal) and who didn't think he had ADD. Next we saw a psychologist, who said Rob was a normal, active little boy. Then we tried an allergist because he craves milk, and then an ear-nose-throat doctor (ENT) because he seems tired a lot and snores. I thought he might have infected adenoids, but he doesn't.

Then we saw a child-development specialist who knew something about sensory problems. He didn't do a formal evaluation but could tell that Rob had an immature, underreactive vestibular system with delays in auditory and visual processing. He gave us specific suggestions for activities to do at home, but they didn't work well because Rob didn't cooperate. Since home therapy wasn't working, we then tested Rob for ADD (negative).

Finally, a neighbor gave me the name of an OT who did a formal evaluation. At three and a half, he was diagnosed with SPD. It was a double relief to have Rob's problem identified and to learn that therapy really helps! After four sessions with her, she feels that with a few months of therapy, Rob has good potential to benefit from OT and that his "nerve problem" will be repaired, and then managing his behavior will be easier.

The pediatrician feels the therapy won't change anything and suggests using more discipline and seeing a child psychologist. But we have already begun to see results and *want to continue the occupational therapy for as long as the OT feels it is necessary. I am hoping we are on the right track.*

This is so unlike anything I have ever been through. This is so hard for me. I am a very "up" person with lots of friends who call me for advice, and for the first time in my adult life I need advice, big time! I've always worked hard to make our lives "perfect," but just getting through the day with Rob has been an accomplishment.

We're not done yet, but we're making progress. Instead of feeling all alone and desperate, now I'm excited and hopeful. When I see Rob's sweet, loving nature emerging, I feel certain we'll restore harmony in our home.

Recognizing When Your Child Needs Professional Help

Ordinarily, growing older means that a child builds upon skills already acquired. A typical child develops the capacity to run after learning to walk, after learning to stand, after learning to creep.

For the out-of-sync child, however, growing older does not always mean getting better at many physical and intellectual tasks, because the basic foundation for efficiently organizing sensory information is shaky.

If growing older does not help, what does? Early intervention! The most appropriate intervention for SPD is OT-SI, which helps the child develop his nervous system.

Before receiving OT-SI or any other form of intervention, the child will need a professional evaluation and a diagnosis. How do you know if an evaluation is necessary?

EIGHT RATIONALIZATIONS THAT PREVENT RECOGNIZING SPD

At least eight rationalizations prevent some people from recognizing SPD and thus seeking a diagnosis. Educators and therapists often hear these comments.

1) **"Looks like ADHD, sounds like ADHD, must be ADHD."** Symptoms of SPD may look like symptoms of several other problems (see chapter 3).

2) **"Never heard of it, so it can't be important."** Many pediatricians, teachers, and other early-childhood experts are unfamiliar with SPD and unable to explain it to parents. Fortunately, it is beginning to be widely acknowledged as more research studies and books in layperson's terms reach the general public.

3) **"Not my kid!"** Even when parents do learn something about SPD, they may be reluctant to believe that it affects their child. People do not go looking for answers if they are in denial that a problem exists.

4) **"So what if he's not a rocket scientist? We love him just the way he is."** Accepting a child "where he's at" is great, but sometimes parents are too accepting. They may be satisfied with their child's irregular development, even if their child is not.

5) **"So what if she doesn't do what other kids do? She is advanced for her age."** Parents may think their child's unchildlike behavior signifies that she is "too smart" for play-dough and playgrounds. However, every child needs to be able to play before she is able to succeed at school. The ability to read at the age of five does not guarantee that she has the physical, social, and emotional readiness for kindergarten.

What looks like precocious behavior may indicate, in fact, a neurological problem. Remember Johnny? Johnny pulled himself to a stand in his crib at five months. At nine months, he walked—on tiptoes! His parents thought he was way ahead of other babies until they learned that his tactile overresponsivity drove him to avoid touching the crib sheet and the ground.

The child may skip typical childhood experiences because she cannot do them. It is illuminating to ask oneself what she avoids. The answer may be elusive, for parents may not realize how much moving, touching, and playing matter. This is a common scenario among families in which the child is the eldest or only one. Without another, more organized child to compare with the disorganized one, parents may be unfamiliar with age-appropriate skills.

6) **"He's so smart, so what if he can't tie his shoes?"** Despite having SPD, the child may have many strengths. He may be a math whiz, a dinosaur expert, or a great storyteller. By contrast, the same child may be weak in self-help skills, sports, or handwriting.

Often, the out-of-sync child develops one or two "splinter skills." These are skills that the child works exceedingly hard to master, but they do not help him generalize his learning to accomplish more complex skills.

For example, one of my preschool students learned to play "Frère Jacques" on the xylophone. He was pleased as punch. Unfortunately, that was his only tune. He played it repeatedly and could not be persuaded to try "Old MacDonald," another simple tune. Another child learned to ride a small bicycle at school—a great accomplishment. However, she had no concept of how to apply her skills to a slightly larger bike at home.

When the child is adept in several areas or achieves a splinter skill, parents, teachers, and pediatricians frequently believe that she has no definable problems. They think she is "just lazy" about learning new skills.

7) **"He can do everything well, if he wants to."** The child may have good days, when he is cooperative, calm, and competent, and bad days, when he is furious, fidgety, and frustrated. Because SPD can manifest itself in different ways, at different times, it is easy to be lulled into false confidence that differences are not the problem.

Parents may believe that the child's erratic behavior is a matter of choice. It is not. No child chooses to be disorganized, but the out-of-sync child may be chronically inconsistent in behavior.

8) **"I was like that, too, and I turned out okay."** That may be true—but was your childhood as easy as you might have wished? Wouldn't it be great if your child could move with a little more grace and comfort as she interacts with the world?

THREE VALID REASONS TO SEEK HELP

Still uncertain whether to seek a diagnosis? If so, consider the following criteria.

1) **Does the problem get in the child's way?** The answer is yes if he struggles with "doing what comes naturally": creeping, running, jumping, climbing, talking, listening, hugging, and playing. The answer is also yes if he has low self-esteem. Indeed, low self-esteem is a red flag of SPD. Sometimes the child will be referred to a mental-health professional. But if the underlying neurological problems are not addressed, the child develops only compensatory techniques, at most.

2) **Does the child's problem get in other people's way?** Yes, if it causes behavior that may not bother the child but bothers everyone else. The child may annoy other children when he pushes, may vex his teacher when he fidgets, and may

scare the wits out of his parents when he is reckless—without comprehending why they are always upset with him.

Yes, if the child is an "angel at home," where it is safe, but a "devil on the street," where it is unpredictable and scary. Yes, if he is an angel at school, where he manages to pull himself together, but a demon at home, where he falls apart at the end of the day. When his behavior differs dramatically in different situations, he is sending out signals of distress.

3) Should you listen when a teacher, pediatrician, or friend suggests you seek help? Yes, if they have dealt with many children and can recognize disorganized behavior. While their advice may hurt, it may also confirm what you sense but have been unable to address. Think of it this way: If the automobile technician says your car needs a tune-up because it is not functioning well, you would listen. How about a tune-up for your out-of-sync child?

Documenting Your Child's Behavior

Parents know their child best but often cannot make sense of what they know. Perhaps you're concerned about your child's difficulties, which do not fit into the traditional medical categories of children's illnesses or disabilities. Perhaps the pediatrician cannot identify the problem, either, and says, "Nothing is wrong. Everything will eventually turn out all right."

What should you do?

First, trust your instincts. Then document your observations.

Documentation is a critical part of the process of identifying and addressing your child's needs. Anecdotal evidence is just as important as a professional diagnosis. Jot down observations you have made at home and incidents teachers have noted at school. Armed with specific data, you will be better equipped to notice patterns and to describe your child's difficulties to a doctor or therapist who is familiar with SPD.

Remember Tommy, Vicki, and Paul? (See chapter 1.) Tommy's differences are tactile; Vicki's are vestibular; Paul's are proprioceptive. (These imaginary children have obvious problems. In real life, SPD may be less clear-cut.)

Below are charts that their parents prepared. The first chart for each child documents the "hard times": situations that cause out-of-sync behavior. The second chart documents the "easy times": situations in which Tommy, Vicki, and Paul function well. (Charts for Sebastian, the overactive and awkward sensory craver, would be similar.)

You may wish to make charts, too, and fill them with clues to help you solve the mystery of your beautiful, but bewildering, child.

TOMMY'S TROUBLING TIMES (TACTILE DIFFERENCES)

Because no one seems able to help, Tommy's parents decide to do some detective work. They begin to chart his most difficult moments, hoping to discover patterns that will offer clues about his behavior. Here is their chart:

Behavior	Date Time	Circumstances
Tantrum! Refused to get dressed.	Oct. 10 8:30 am	Says his socks are too tight and he hates his new turtle-neck sweater.
Inconsolable at school.	Oct. 14 10:00 am	Teacher said he was fine until it was time for art project (finger painting).

Behavior	Date Time	Circumstances
Threw plate on kitchen floor.	Oct. 22 noon	I thought he'd like cottage cheese (instead of yogurt) for a change. Wrong!
Screamed in grocery store. Threw a grape at friendly old lady.	Nov. 23 4:30 pm	Day before Thanksgiving. Noisy, crowded store. Old lady (stranger) tousled his hair.
Single-handedly destroyed toys at Santa's Workshop.	Dec. 18 2:00 pm	Excited by toys in the department store and couldn't keep his hands off them. Out of control, like a bull in a china shop.

Interpretation of Tommy's Troubling Times

Unrelated as the charted notations seem, they indicate a pattern of tactile dysfunction. Let's look at the incidents one by one.

First incident: Tommy fusses over his clothes because he is uncomfortable in high collars and bumpy socks. He is not purposely ornery. He simply cannot explain why certain textures are irritating. His poorly regulated tactile system is the culprit, telling him on a subconscious level that his clothes are threatening his sense of well-being. His mother remarks, "The person who invents the truly seamless sock will make a fortune!"

Second incident: Tommy is inconsolable at school because of finger painting. The teacher, believing that she offers pleasurable activities to her students, is mystified and urges Tommy to participate. He hates the thought of wet, messy hands, feels like a failure, and wishes the teacher would leave him alone. The scene escalates into a very unhappy situation.

Third incident: Tommy makes a scene at lunch. He has

eating problems, for his mouth is overly sensitive to the food textures. If you remember the first time you put a raw oyster in your mouth, you can sympathize! Tommy will eat yogurt because it is familiar and safe. Lumpy cottage cheese, however, is not safe. Tommy cannot explain that his defensive tactile system is sending up alert signals, so he hurls his plate down.

Fourth incident: In the supermarket, Tommy bops a friendly woman on the head with a grape. Why does he lash out, making his mother wish she could just abandon him and the Thanksgiving turkey and go home to weep? The answer is simple: To Tommy, the woman is a threat. She is unfamiliar, and she makes the "mistake" of patting him on the head.

For all of us, our heads are extra-sensitive to unexpected light touch. Most of us react instantly to light touch in order to protect the body parts we need for survival. Because Tommy is more sensitive than most, he reacts with what we might consider an excessive response.

Fifth incident: Tommy tears into the toys at Santa's Workshop. Whereas others his age may be satisfied to look at and maybe caress the toys with a discriminative touch, Tommy "attacks" them. An aspect of his out-of-sync touch system requires him to manhandle objects in order to learn about them. Poor Tommy! He wreaks havoc in Santa's Workshop because he wants to know (and, of course, own) all the toys.

In summary, Tommy has SPD in his tactile system, involving overresponsivity and poor discrimination.

TOMMY'S TERRIFIC TIMES

Noting Tommy's out-of-sync behavior gives only half the picture. Tommy's parents also chart his terrific times, when he is more positively in sync.

Behavior	Date Time	Circumstances
Fell asleep easily.	Oct. 11 7:30 pm	Asked for a back rub: "Daddy do it, not Mommy." (Art was pleased; usually Tommy prefers me to his dad.) "Down, not up!" Art rubbed his back hard with firm, downward strokes and gave ten tight bear hugs for more deep pressure. Then Tommy asked Art to put him to bed—a first!
Enjoyed bath and again fell asleep easily.	Oct. 12 7:30 pm	Two good ideas: having Tommy help get the water temperature "just right" (lukewarm), and using Art's rubbing technique, first with a washcloth, then with a sponge. "More, Mommy, more!" The rubbing relaxed him.
Had a great day at school.	Oct. 15 9:00 am– noon	I told his teacher that he likes rubdowns, so she tried the "people sandwich" game. He was the "baloney," squished between two gym mats ("bread"). Loved it. Rest of the day went well.
Ate lunch without complaint.	Oct. 15 12:30 pm	Gave him pureed soup—no lumps. He chowed it down and had a second bowl. Why did it take me so long to realize he will eat only smooth food?
Actually enjoyed trip to grocery store.	Nov. 30 3:00 pm	Went to supermarket that has miniature carts for kids. He liked pushing one, loaded with potatoes and apples, and was a great helper. Good idea to take him when store isn't crowded.

Behavior	Date Time	Circumstances
Sat on kitchen floor and kept me company for an hour while I baked.	Jan. 5 2:00 pm	His teacher said he enjoyed handling dried beans in the big bin. (He avoids the bin when it has water or sand.) I filled a dishpan with peas, pinto beans, and lentils and gave him some measuring cups and a scoop. He busily measured and poured beans, chatting away. He said, "This is fun work."

Interpretation of Tommy's Terrific Times

First incident: Firm, predictable touch has always comforted Tommy. He asks for a back rub with downward strokes—the way hair grows. (Upward strokes "ruffle his feathers" and "rub him the wrong way.") He prefers his father's deep pressure to his mother's gentler caresses. Firm, soothing pressure suppresses his overresponsivity and prepares him for sleep.

Second incident: Tommy's mother invites him to help adjust the water temperature before he gets in the bath. He likes having some control rather than being plunged into water that is "too hot!" or "too cold!" That night he climbs in willingly. Also, she takes a cue from her husband and rubs Tommy's back and limbs firmly with a washcloth and sponge, instead of sprinkling him clean. He relaxes, and the result is another pleasant bedtime.

Third incident: The teacher tries a deep-pressure activity at school, with much success. Tommy enjoys being pounded with "mustard" and crawled over by his classmates. Therapeutic and fun, the "people sandwich" activity also helps him interact with his peers.

Fourth incident: Tommy cannot tolerate lumps in his food. When his mother prepares soup with a smooth texture, he likes it.

Fifth incident: Tommy likes pushing the little grocery cart. He can get a good grip on the smooth handlebar, which does not irritate his hands. The deep muscle work of pushing something with resistance feels good. Also, Tommy's mother is paying more attention to his fear of crowds. She notes that going to the store when it is quiet makes the outing enjoyable.

Sixth incident: Tommy likes handling the dried beans because they are not sticky, and he becomes engrossed in his play. Comparing notes about his behavior, his mother and teacher can strategize ways to provide him with successful tactile experiences at home and school.

VICKI'S VICISSITUDES (VESTIBULAR DIFFERENCES)

Vicki's parents take notes about their child's inconsistent behavior:

Behavior	Date Time	Circumstances
Strolling to corner mailbox, stumbled and fell. Cried, "So tired. Carry me!"	June 4 9:30 am	After a long night's sleep and good breakfast, why should she be so limp? But sometimes, by the end of the day, she's raring to go!
Refused to let me leave her at Ellen's birthday party. Once the games began, she became wound up and uncontrollable.	June 9 2:30 pm	So excited about the party, until we arrived. The whole class was invited to play tag and relay races. I was the only mom who had to stay, and Vicki was the only child who didn't play. When she finally left my side, the activities really wound her up. She was in everybody's face, shouting, pushing, and running wildly. Everyone was in tears. We left early.

Behavior	Date Time	Circumstances
Fell apart at the playground. Tantrum lasted twenty minutes.	July 3 2:30 pm	Yesterday she loved the play-ground; today she hated it. Same place, same time, same weather, but different child! All I did was spin her a few times on the tire swing. Usually, she loves the tire swing.
When we pointed to the moon, she kept looking at our fingers rather than the sky.	Sept. 4 9:30 pm	Up later than usual. Other kids at neighborhood picnic excited about the bright moon and stars. Vicki didn't understand what she was supposed to be looking at.

Interpretation of Vicki's Vicissitudes

First incident: Vicki's early-morning fatigue is a symptom of low muscle tone; she has a loose and limp body. A short excursion to the corner mailbox requires more energy than she can muster at the moment. Also, her trunk is unstable and she has poor postural responses, poor balance, and poor motor coordination. Her mother notes, however, that in the evening, Vicki is energetic after experiencing intense movement.

Second incident: New situations distress Vicki. Difficulty controlling her movements causes her to be emotionally inse-cure, so she clings to her mother. Poor coordination and poor motor planning hinder her ability to socialize effectively with her classmates. Her need for vigorous movement is keen, but when she eventually joins in the games, she goes overboard, crashing and bumping into the other children.

Third incident: Knowing that Vicki often enjoys the tire swing, her mother thinks she will enjoy it even more with a little help to make it spin faster. Vicki cannot tolerate the unexpected passive movement, however. Vicki hates being on the tire swing when someone else moves it; she likes it only when she is in control.

Fourth incident: Looking at the moon poses another problem. Vicki's eye movements are not well coordinated. Because her eyes do not work well together, she has poor eye teaming and poor depth perception. She looks at her parents' wagging fingers, within her visual range, and seems unable to gaze beyond her immediate space.

In summary, Vicki is underresponsive to vestibular sensations. Associated problems are low muscle tone, dyspraxia and postural challenges, and poor ocular control.

VICKI'S VICTORIES

Vicki's parents also take notes about successful situations.

Behavior	Date Time	Circumstances
Spent 5 minutes standing on her head. Afterward, was calm and attentive.	June 6 8:00 pm	Tried to get Vicki into bed to listen to a story, but she was revved up, walking in circles. Finally, she went to the corner and got into an upside-down position. I read the story and she listened quietly. Then she came back to earth, climbed into bed, and fell instantly asleep.
At park, swung for 45 minutes! Bubbly, bright, and talkative all afternoon.	July 2 2:30 pm	First, she lay on the swing, tummy down, and pushed with her toes. Second, she sat on the swing and asked me to push her for a very long time. Third, she spun herself around on the tire swing. She wasn't dizzy, but I was, just watching!

Behavior	Date Time	Circumstances
Tipped to and fro on a makeshift teeter-totter. Later, seemed more in sync than usual.	July 12 2:30 pm	Vicki joined other kids as they played on the teeter-totter they had made with a plywood board over railroad timber. She rocked from side to side and enjoyed the jolt whenever the edge of the board hit the ground. She had fun finding different ways to balance.
Played happily (for a change!) with other kids at the lake.	Aug. 1 4:00 pm	Instead of throwing and catching the ball, she had fun sitting and lying on it. When she fell off onto the grass, she laughed. The other kids were interested in her ideas, and they all took turns. It's great to see her playing with others!

Interpretation of Vicki's Victories

First incident: Positioning herself upside down, feet in the air, is a form of self-therapy. Although this position seems odd, it helps regulate Vicki's inefficient processing. Through her inner ear she is receiving useful information about the pull of gravity.

Second incident: Vicki enjoys swinging in different ways for an unusually long time. When she decides how to move and for how long, she is actively engaging in self-therapy. Hanging upside down provides one kind of intense vestibular intake that her brain craves. Swaying gently back and forth, a form of linear movement through space, is soothing. Spinning on the tire swing, a form of rotary movement, also helps regulate her vestibular system.

The fact that she does not get dizzy when she spins indicates that her vestibular system is out of sync. Normally, prolonged spinning would make a person feel woozy, but it makes Vicki feel wonderful.

After swinging, she is chatty and vivacious. The activities have aroused the language centers of her brain. Like all children, she has a lot to say; unlike most children, she often has trouble getting the words out. When she "primes the pump," the words begin to flow.

Third incident: Rocking from side to side is a form of linear motion called oscillation. Like swinging, it organizes Vicki's vestibular system. She likes the jolting sensation when the board strikes the ground. The jolts arouse her in a positive way by sending extra messages to her joints and muscles. When she directs her own play, she plays with purpose and good attention.

Fourth incident: Tossing a beach ball is too hard due to Vicki's poor motor skills. However, she enjoys a different challenge: maintaining her balance while sitting on the ball. Every child has an inner drive to resist gravity. Sometimes all the child needs is the right equipment in the right place at the right time! When the other children join her game, Vicki's self-confidence soars and she is able to play with them happily.

PAUL'S PROBLEMS (PROPRIOCEPTIVE DIFFERENCES)

Paul's parents prepare this chart as they look for patterns:

Behavior	Date Time	Circumstances
Walked into a telephone pole and required three stitches.	July 9 3:30 pm	Leaving ice cream parlor, Paul was paying attention to his cone, not to where he was going. So exasperating and frustrating!

Behavior	Date Time	Circumstances
Picked up Granny's china figurine, then smashed it to smithereens when he set it down.	Aug. 2 8:00 pm	Maybe he was tired after long trip getting to Granny's, but even when he's rested he's clumsy. Granny's unhappiness worsened the situation. She wasn't angry at him, just sad. He was inconsolable.
Trying to play catch with a beach ball, he missed it every time.	Aug. 4 noon	Paul either lunges at the ball at the wrong time or swats it away. His younger cousins are so mean and say, "Baby! Baby! Don't you even know how to catch a ball?"
At the restaurant, spilled his milk on the tablecloth and his good clothes.	Labor Day 6:30 pm	Sometimes Paul can't seem to manage getting milk into his mouth. Even though the waitress was a sweetheart, Paul was distraught.
Late for first day of fifth grade because he had a fit buttoning his new shirt.	Sept 6 8:30 to 9:30 am	First he resisted wearing the shirt and then buttoned it incorrectly, saying, "They made it wrong. I never do anything right." He works so hard to do the simplest things.

Interpretation of Paul's Problems

First incident: Paul bumps into a pole because eating the cone requires his full attention. He really cannot chew and walk at the same time. His mother's frustration is nothing compared to Paul's!

Second incident: Paul misjudges the weight of Granny's figurine. Of course Granny is upset. It is hard to understand that poor control over the force he puts into every movement causes his carelessness.

Third incident: It is about as easy for Paul to catch a beach ball as it is for most of us to capture a butterfly. He has trouble moving through space, coordinating his arms and legs, and anticipating the impact of the ball. No wonder his cousins are "so mean!" They do not like to play with him because they cannot predict what he will do and how he will do it. They notice his jerky movements and consider him a "jerk."

Fourth incident: The outing to a restaurant is a disaster. When Paul picks up a glass that feels unfamiliar, the sensations from his muscles cannot tell him how much effort to exert. The glass of milk flies through the air, and Paul, once again, makes a mess.

Fifth incident: Buttoning a stiff shirt is hard for Paul. Normal first-day-of-school anxiety, plus Mother's urgings to move faster, plus his clumsiness, add up to Paul's deep despair. Because he moves inefficiently, he has low self-esteem. When he cries "I never do anything right," he really believes what he says.

In summary, Paul's main problem is poor discrimination of proprioceptive, tactile, and vestibular sensations, along with sensory-based motor differences.

PAUL'S POSITIVES

Paul's parents also record his positive experiences:

Behavior	Date Time	Circumstances
Pleased to write a brief note to Granny before our trip.	July 28 3:30 pm	Before starting to write, Paul cracked all his knuckles and squeezed his fingers. Explained, "My hands work better when I do this." Wrote without breaking the pencil point!

Behavior	Date Time	Circumstances
Loved playing Granny's "posture game."	Aug. 4 10:00 am	Granny challenged him to walk around with a cookbook on his head longer than she can. Paul "won" and earned a trip to the baseball card shop. She makes him "shape up." He adores her.
Enjoyed a tug-of-war game on the beach.	Aug. 7 noon	We had to play a silly game of tug-of-war with cousins to prove that our family is just as strong as theirs. Paul loved it! Said, "It's awesome to be on a team." He's developing a competitive streak this summer. Astonishing.
Helped wash Ron's car; then volunteered to wash mine, too.	Dec. 28 2:00 pm	Paul volunteered to lug buckets of water from the house. He can lift a really heavy weight! Enjoyed helping Ron sponge and dry the car. He said, "I bet you're glad to have a son like me." It's a joy to hear him say that. We need to assign him more chores.

Interpretation of Paul's Positives

First incident: Paul is "waking up" his writing muscles when he cracks his knuckles and squeezes his fingers. He needs extra stimulation in his hands to manipulate a pencil. His mother remarks that after this exercise he does not break the pencil point as he usually does.

Second incident: Granny's technique to improve Paul's posture is therapeutically sound. The weight of the book compresses the muscles in his neck and shoulders and gives him extrasensory information. He stands up straighter, in an adaptive behavior to resist gravity. Granny's technique is also psychologically sound. She guesses correctly that he will accept her challenge because it is fun and not too demanding. Succeeding boosts his self-esteem, and tomorrow he may try a bigger challenge—like a dictionary!

Third incident: Pulling the rope organizes Paul's proprioceptive system. He enjoys the tug-of-war because stretching his muscles feels good. He also likes being on a team where everyone is working together and no one can be singled out as the "loser." Like all children, Paul has the inner drive to use his muscles effectively, but he is not a self-starter. He does not know how to engage in activities that benefit his proprioceptive system unless the opportunity is literally put into his hands.

Fourth incident: Paul stretches his muscles vigorously when he hoists water buckets, squeezes the sponge, and towels the car. This activity energizes him, and he's ready to wash another car. His mother's plan to give him more chores will help Paul, for every child needs to feel useful.

Diagnosing the Problem

Consider the adage "When you hear hoofbeats, look for horses, not zebras." Documenting your child's responses will help you locate those "horses," the specific situations causing out-of-sync behavior.

Maybe you can spot the problem clearly. Maybe you cannot. What should you do? Where do you start? You have three choices:

1) You could take the "wait-and-see" approach—but please don't! It is not advisable to sit back and wait for your out-of-sync child to catch up, if his differences get in his way every day. Possibly, with time, he will

function better—but probably his life will just get harder. Why take a chance when getting help now may make a tremendous difference in his coping skills?

2) You could enrich your child's sensory way of life. Joining forces with the teacher, you could develop a home-and-school program that will help your child strengthen his skills. (See chapters 11 and 12.)

3) You could seek specialist(s) who will either screen your child for possible risk factors or do a full evaluation. (Screenings and evaluations are described below.) Ask the pediatrician first for a referral to a specialist. If the doctor resists this idea for some reason, try one of the support systems listed below.

WHERE TO TURN FOR SUPPORT

Everything we can learn about our children's development makes us better parents and teachers. Whether you are certain or uncertain that your child has SPD, gathering information about his strengths and weaknesses will affect how you educate, discipline, and even regard him.

If you live in the United States, to get a screening or an evaluation, start with either early intervention services for a child age three or younger, or your local school district for a child older than three. These free resources are available under IDEA 04.[1]

If Your Child Is Under Three

Each state in the United States has a system of early intervention services for infants and toddlers (birth through age two) who have developmental delays—or certain disabilities that are likely to result in developmental delays—and their families. The child is eligible for referral and screening but is eligible for evaluation only if the screening indicates that a disability is suspected, and then is eligible for intervention only if he or she meets different state requirements.

Evaluation to determine whether your child is eligible for early intervention services is free of charge. You will be found eligible for services if your child is determined, through evaluation, to have developmental delays in one or more of five areas of development (cognitive, physical, communication, social/emotional, or adaptive development) or to be at high risk for developing a delay due to a diagnosed physical or mental condition. If your child's sensory processing differences impact any of the five areas of development, he or she may meet the eligibility requirements for early intervention services.

If the evaluation finds your child eligible, an Individualized Family Service Plan (IFSP) is developed. The IFSP outlines the supports and services to help you as a family best support your child's development. The IFSP includes service coordination and may also include occupational therapy, physical therapy, speech-and-language, and other services, depending on need. Services through early intervention often occur in the home or sometimes in a community center. These services are free or at low cost, depending on the policies of your state.

If you have concerns about your child's development, you can ask your pediatrician for a referral to early intervention services, or you may contact your local early intervention program directly and ask to have your child evaluated. You can find information about early intervention services in your state online by searching for your state name and the term "early intervention."

If Your Child Is Three or Older

If your child is three or older, your local school district will be the place to start.

Eligibility for services through the public schools is all about getting an education. If your child's sensory processing differences impact her ability to make effective progress in school, he or she may be able to receive services through the public schools at no cost to the family. Eligibility for special education services varies from state to state. Therefore, understanding your state's requirements is very important. This information helps parents have realistic expectations and prevents frustration for parents and schools.

Here's the deal: If your child is eligible, the school is required to develop an Individualized Education Program (IEP), including supports and services to ensure that your child is provided a free appropriate public education (FAPE). If your child is ineligible, the school is not required to provide services.

The IDEA 04 requires schools to provide special education and related services to eligible students. But not every child with SPD qualifies. To be eligible, your child's school performance must be adversely impacted by one of thirteen educational disability categories, including specific learning disability, other health impairment, autism, serious emotional disturbance, intellectual disability, hearing impairment, deafness, speech or language impairments, vision impairment/blindness, orthopedic impairment, traumatic brain injury, deaf-blindness, or multiple disabilities.

The educational disability category of "other health impairment" includes chronic or acute health problems (one of which is ADHD) that adversely affect the child's educational performance. In some situations, SPD may be considered an other health impairment, described in the law as "limited strength, vitality or alertness, including a heightened alertness to environmental stimuli that result in limited alertness with respect to the educational environment." The caveat here is that SPD is not always acknowledged or recognized as a health problem, in large part because it is not included in the *DSM-5*.

If ineligible under IDEA 04, the child with SPD may be eligible under Section 504 of the Rehabilitation Act of 1973, the antidiscrimination law.[2] A child is eligible for accommodations (which may include services) when he has a physical or mental impairment that substantially limits one or more major life activities. Major life activities include functions such as caring for oneself, performing manual tasks, walking, seeing, hearing, speaking, breathing, learning, and working.

If the child is ineligible under both IDEA 04 and Section 504, check with these other places:

- Your child's preschool or early childhood center, which may suggest a few local OTs who are familiar with SI treatment and who work well with children.
- Private, nonprofit mental health and social service organizations, which may provide services, often on a sliding scale.
- A multidisciplinary teaching hospital for a full evaluation.
- The occupational therapy department of your local children's hospital.
- STAR Institute, www.sensoryhealth.org, which posts a free online directory of OTs and other professionals who work with individuals with SPD.

WHAT IS A SCREENING?

A screening is a quick and simple procedure during which an OT or other qualified examiner checks whether children have acquired specific skills. Often, groups of children are screened at the same time at schools or early childhood centers.

The purpose of a screening is the early identification of children who may have one or more developmental difficulties: cognitive, physical, speech and language, psychosocial, self-help, or adaptive.

A screening is a short, informal "look-see." It is neither a test nor an in-depth examination. When it suggests that a child may have a problem, parents are notified and encouraged to have the child fully evaluated.

WHAT IS AN EVALUATION?

A formal evaluation is a thorough, individualized examination to look at the whole person and measure his or her skills. The type of professional performing the evaluation depends on the child's presenting problem(s). An occupational therapist is the professional who typically evaluates children with suspected sensory processing problems. Other professionals may also be involved, such as a developmental optometrist (eye doctor), audiologist (specialist in problems related to hearing loss), speech/language pathologist, pediatrician, psychologist, special educator, and/or social worker. If the child has severe SPD, a multidisciplinary team composed of several of these professionals may be necessary and would provide a more comprehensive report.

One part of the evaluation is a questionnaire that parents complete, such as a medical, sensory-motor, developmental, or family history. To see a sample sensory-motor history questionnaire by Sharon Cermak, EdD, et al., see www.out-of-sync-child.com. Sometimes teachers are asked to fill out questionnaires, too. Your answers will help the OT or other professionals assess your child, as patterns of behavior since birth may confirm clinical observations.

Providing information about your child will help you, too. Indeed, after completing a sensory-motor questionnaire, one mother noted, "We've been puzzled by our four-year-old's cautiousness, language delay, picky eating, and sensitivity to touch, but we never understood the connection. Now the pieces are beginning to fit!"

Another part of the evaluation is the child's visit with the OT in a hospital, clinic, office, school, or your home. The evaluation is based on standardized tests,[3] when possible, and structured observations and analysis of your child's strengths and limitations. In addition, observations in a natural (nontesting) setting, such as your home or your child's day care or school, are also important to assess your child's actual observed abilities in a familiar setting. Depending on how much testing is required, the evaluation will take from one hour to several hours, spread over several days.

The OT considers the child's strengths and limitations. Where, when, how often, and with what intensity do problems occur? How long has the child exhibited the problem behavior? What is the age level at which the child performs? What is happening at home or school that may be affecting his ability to function? What situations bring out the worst and the best in him? Why, in the OT's opinion, is the child out of sync?

The crucial question is "What kind of SPD is this?" Is it tactile overresponsivity? Postural, bilateral, or ocular difficulties?

Poor auditory discrimination? Dr. Ayres and her followers have always insisted on determining the child's sensory needs so that treatment can be specific.

After careful consideration, the therapist writes a detailed report and confers with parents to help them interpret the results. (Sometimes a doctor will make the diagnosis based on the qualified examiner's report.) Often, the report is informative. If you receive one that is difficult to understand, call the professional back for a better explanation. She wants to help you, not confuse you.

Therapy may not be indicated if a child is simply immature. Abundant sensory-motor experiences over time may be the late bloomer's best treatment. The professional may suggest a sensory-enriched life at home with specific activities that you can do as a family or that the child's teacher can implement at school. These activities are enjoyable for everybody and help all children strengthen their neurological skills.

If, however, a problem is evident, the professional will recommend direct therapy sessions. If you decide to enroll your child, you will not be obligated to stick with the professional who conducted the evaluation. Finding the right therapist is important because a good fit between therapist and child will affect your child's progress.

The Occupational Therapist's Evaluation
An occupational therapist will usually evaluate the child in her office. The evaluation is ordinarily a pleasant experience. While costs vary, expect to spend several hundred dollars. This will be money well spent, and it may be covered by health insurance.

Sensory processing is just one of several areas the OT is qualified to address. Here are some of the underlying areas an OT investigates as they impact a child's ability to participate in daily life activities or "occupations":

- Fine- and gross-motor developmental levels
- Visual-motor integration (doing puzzles or copying shapes)
- Visual discrimination
- Neuromuscular control (balance and posture)
- Responses to sensory stimulation (tactile, vestibular, and proprioceptive)
- Bilateral coordination
- Praxis (motor planning)

The OT may identify needs in other areas as well, such as challenges with attention, a possible language delay, or an auditory, visual, or emotional problem. If she finds that your child has difficulties in these areas, she may refer you to another professional for further evaluation.

WHO PAYS FOR TREATMENT?

Although therapy may be clearly indicated for your child, not all health insurance policies cover the expense. It may help you to get coverage if your pediatrician puts it into writing that therapy is a medical necessity. However, as mentioned earlier in this chapter, sensory differences are not always acknowledged or recognized as a health problem.

The reason is that SPD is not yet included in all of the publications of diagnostic classification systems, such as the *DSM-5*.

However, SPD is now included in the *Diagnostic Classification of Mental Health and Developmental Disorders of Infancy and Early Childhood (DC:0-5)*.[4] As formal recognition of the disorder grows, so will support for multidisciplinary research and availability of services for children and their families.

Whether or not your child has been identified as being learning disabled, a pronounced problem with educational functioning is sometimes considered to be a sufficient criterion for funding.

If, in addition to SPD, your child has significant medical, physical, and developmental problems, then she is eligible to receive services. If your child is enrolled in a special-education class in a public school, then related services such as occupational therapy, physical therapy, and speech/language therapy may be part of the free educational program when your child's school team determines these services are required in order for your child to progress in school.

If a child is eligible under IDEA 04 or Section 504, the public school district is legally responsible for developing an IEP or a Section 504 accommodation plan and providing the special education and related services and accommodations included in these documents. If the child is not eligible, parents may still request that teachers and schools provide accommodations for the child, although the teachers and the school district are not required to do so.

It is important to understand that the services provided by the public school may not address all of your child's SPD differences because they are focused specifically on ensuring that your child is able to participate and progress in academic work at school. In some situations, parents may pursue OT-SI outside of school and in addition to what the public school is providing in order to address all of the child's SPD-related needs.

Otherwise, paying for therapy is up to you.

So—you must weigh the expense versus the benefits.

One benefit is what a therapist offers: her training and expertise, her therapeutic equipment, and her ability to provide experiences that your child cannot get elsewhere. Another, most important, benefit is knowing that you are acting in your child's best interest. By investing in treatment now, you forestall problems that may later cause greater pain and more expensive therapy.

You will have many decisions to make, but should you get intervention for your child, you will probably see an enormous change in his behavior, his feelings, his skills, and your family life.

Different Therapies, Different Approaches

After an evaluation, the next step is to arrange for treatment. The most beneficial treatment for SPD is OT-SI, occupational therapy using a sensory integration framework.

OCCUPATIONAL THERAPY

Occupational therapy, an allied health profession, encompasses evaluation, assessment, treatment, and consultation. OT is the use of purposeful activity to maximize the independence and the maintenance of the health of an individual who is limited by a physical injury or illness, cognitive impairment, a psychosocial dysfunction, a mental illness, a developmental or learning disability, or an adverse environmental condition. For a child, purposeful activities include swinging, climbing, jumping, buttoning, drawing, and writing. Such activities are the child's "occupation."

The specific goals of OT-SI are to improve and harmonize the person's relationships, self-regulation, and sensory integration. According to Virginia Spielmann, executive director of the STAR Institute, "The end goal . . . is more than a mere absence of dysfunctional sensory processing and integration; it is psychological well-being or 'flourishing.'"[5]

The Occupational Therapist

An occupational therapist (also abbreviated as OT) is a healthcare professional who has received a baccalaureate, master's, or doctoral degree after completing a course of study, plus internship experience, in the biological, physical, medical, and behavioral sciences. (Since 2007, all new OT candidates must earn a postbaccalaureate degree.) Coursework includes neurology, anatomy, orthopedics, psychology, and psychiatry.

The OT may work with your child individually or in a group, at school, in a clinic, hospital, community mental health center, or your home. The ideal OT is one who specializes in pediatrics and who has received additional postgraduate training in sensory integration theory and treatment.

Under the guidance of a therapist, the child actively takes in movement and touch information in playful, meaningful, and natural ways that help his brain modulate these fundamental neural messages. The child responds favorably to SI treatment, because his nervous system is pliable and changeable. Therapy teaches the child to succeed—and he loves it!

Activities the OT May Provide

Every child is different, so the sequence and kinds of activity that an occupational therapist provides for your child will be individualized. She will design a program based on his particular needs, going back in his system to where early skills have been mastered. Following his lead, she will guide him through "just-right challenges" that affect his central nervous system and challenge his ability to respond successfully to sensory stimuli in an organized way.

For instance, your child may have difficulty jumping, climbing, pedaling tricycles, and getting dressed. These problems cannot be "fixed" by teaching him specifically how to jump, climb, pedal, and put on a jacket, when the underlying problem is SPD. He does not need jumping lessons but opportunities to integrate all sensations. With her appealing equipment and professional knowledge, a qualified therapist can weave art and science together to offer these opportunities.

Here is a small sampling of activities that an OT may provide:

- To reduce tactile overresponsivity—having arms and legs rubbed with differently textured sponges and cloths
- To improve tactile discrimination—finding hidden toys by manipulating a ball of therapeutic putty
- To develop better body awareness and improve postural security—swinging prone in a special swing suspended from the ceiling, in order to experience specific movement sensations
- To improve balance—lying or sitting on large, inflated therapy balls
- To improve bilateral coordination—using a rolling pin with both hands to bat at a ball hanging from the ceiling, while lying prone

- To improve motor planning—moving through obstacle courses
- To improve fine-motor skills—playing with magnets to build up the muscles of the hand to stabilize loose joints
- To improve extension against the pull of gravity—riding across the floor, or riding headfirst down a ramp, while lying prone on a scooter
- To improve flexion—clinging to a cylindrical swing that is suspended from the ceiling
- To reduce gravitational insecurity—swinging gently on a flat glider swing; jumping on a bounce pad
- To improve ocular control and visual discrimination—playing games with beanbags, balloons, and suspended balls

The most important factor that will determine the success of therapy is the child's own inner drive to explore and learn from the environment. The child's motivation to spin on a swing, to touch certain textures, or to be gently pressed between two gym mats tells the therapist what the child's nervous system seeks.

According to Dr. Ayres, "Sensations that make a child happy tend to be integrating."[6] When the child is actively involved in his own therapy, he becomes more organized, he has fun, and he feels in sync.

OTHER TYPES OF THERAPY

While the child with SPD will benefit most from OT-SI, therapies that support coexisting difficulties will also help. A few are mentioned here. (Note: SPD is a neurological problem, but most neurologists are not trained to evaluate it in children, and they do not provide SI therapy.)

Physical Therapy

Physical therapy is a health profession devoted to improving an individual's physical abilities. It involves activities that strengthen the child's muscular control and motor coordination, especially of his large muscles. Sometimes by using physical agents such as massage, whirlpool baths, or ultrasound, physical therapists help the child get his muscles ready for voluntary movement. Some physical therapists receive additional training in sensory integration theory and treatment. See https://aptaapps.apta.org//APTAPTDirectory/FindAPTDirectory.aspx to find a therapist. Also see www.ndta.org about the multidisciplinary, holistic, neurodevelopmental approach used by PTs, OTs, and SLPs for clients who have difficulty controlling movement as a result of neurological challenges.

Speech-and-Language Therapy

Speech-and-language therapy includes activities designed to meet specific goals for the child. The child may require help with speech skills, such as pronouncing "l," "k," or "sh" sounds; monitoring the pitch of his voice; and strengthening oral-motor control in his mouth muscles. He may benefit from activities designed to expand his language skills, such as retelling stories, conversing, and playing games to develop memory. He may need help with social pragmatics—that is, using language and gestures to interact with others. Also, as many children with SPD are highly selective eaters or problem feeders, therapy with an OT and a speech-and-language pathologist (SLP) trained in oral-motor and feeding issues may be very helpful. See www .asha.org and www.sosapproachtofeeding.com.

Vision Therapy

Vision therapy (VT) is a set of procedures, performed under the direction of a developmental/behavioral optometrist, to correct or enhance the skills necessary for proper vision. A developmental vision exam includes an evaluation of eye health as well as eyesight and how vision, touch, hearing, movement, and other senses work together. After the evaluation, the optometrist may recommend VT, which could include prescription lenses, prisms, sensory-motor activities, and even computer-based programs to enhance eye-motor control, visual discrimination, and eye-hand coordination. Much more than just eye exercises, VT helps the child integrate visual information with other sensory input. This treatment often helps a child's eyes and body function in sync and can prevent and remediate learning-related visual problems. See www.covd.org, www.oep.org, and www.optometrists.org.

Auditory Training

Auditory training is a method of sound stimulation designed to improve a person's listening and communicative skills, learning capabilities, motor coordination, body awareness, and self-esteem. Several times a week, the child/adult listens to music and voices filtered through special headphones, engages in specific visual and balance activities, and may participate in voice work. Therapy helps the ear to attend to and discriminate among sounds, the vestibular system to integrate sensory messages of balance and posture, and the person to become more focused, centered, and organized. See www.tomatis.com, www

.berardaitwebsite.com, www.VitalLinks.net, www.advanced brain.com, and www.integratedlistening.com to learn about different programs.

Chiropractic

Chiropractic is the philosophy, art, and science of detecting and correcting subluxation in the human body. Subluxation is a partial dislocation or abnormal movement of a bone in a joint. Chiropractic helps children with SPD by specifically addressing the structure and function of the nerves, muscles, and joints controlling posture and movement that influence our ability to interact with our environment. Some chiropractic approaches successfully integrate sensory-motor, language, cognitive, and other therapies to balance both sides of the brain. See www .icpa4kids.com.

CranioSacral Therapy

CranioSacral Therapy (CST) is a gentle method of evaluating and enhancing the function of the craniosacral system (the membranes and cerebrospinal fluid that protect the brain and spinal cord). CST involves light-touch manipulation of the bones in the skull, sacrum, and coccyx to correct an imbalance that can adversely affect the development of the brain and spinal cord and can result in sensory, motor, and neurological dysfunction. CST is used by a variety of health-care professionals. See www.upledger.com.

Hippotherapy

Hippotherapy means "treatment with the help of the horse." Occupational, physical, and speech therapists use the horse as a modality to improve the posture, movement, neuromotor function, and sensory processing of people with disabilities. The movement of the horse, with traditional therapy intervention, influences muscle tone, encourages muscle action, and improves vestibular reactions, sensory-motor integration, and midline postural control. See www.americanhippotherapy association.org.

Nutritional Therapy

Good nutrition is essential for development, efficient maintenance, and functioning, optimum activity level, and resistance to infection and disease. A nutritionist can help a person with dietary deficiencies achieve balance in carbohydrates, fats, protein, vitamins, minerals, and water. See www.kellydorfman .com and www.mariarickerthong.com.

Supportive Counseling

Behavioral therapy helps the child deal with problematical symptoms and ways of behaving. Play therapy promotes the child's social/emotional development. Family therapy helps the child, parents, and siblings become a healthier unit. These are examples of therapies that recruit the logical, thinking brain to impact the body, behavioral expressions, and emotional states. Therapists include clinical psychologists, licensed clinical social workers, and child psychiatrists. (Psychotherapy is sometimes appropriate to deal with the social/emotional effects of SPD, such as depression or problems with self-image and behavior, but it does not deal with the underlying causes.) See www.icdl.com and www.profectum.org.

Supportive Community-Based Activities

In addition to therapies, community-based activities can be considered therapeutic as they help children develop physical and cognitive skills, a sense of self, and social relationships. Many elementary-school-aged and older children enjoy martial arts, such as karate and tae kwon do (www.ataonline.com/ata _karateforkids), which develop strength, flexibility, and endurance. Music therapy (www.musictherapy.org) and art therapy (www.arttherapy.org) are other possible treatments. Virginia Spielmann at STAR Institute suggests nature walks and rambles, wall climbing and rock scrambles, yoga, dance, and rebounder/trampoline exercise. She sees emerging evidence, also, about the benefits of massage such as Qigong Sensory Treatment (www.qsti.org).

Bringing Therapist and Child Together

Before the first session with the OT (or other therapist), you will want to prepare your child. You can say, "Today you'll meet someone who will help you get stronger. She has great toys and games to play. Her place is like a gym where you will do things that feel good. I think you'll have lots of fun."

Emphasizing that therapy will be fun is important. Many children with SPD do not have much fun. They wish they could but simply do not know how.

When you think and speak positively about therapy, you help make it work for your child. You reassure your child that this is not punishment or something to feel defensive about. The child may blame himself for being frequently clumsy or tired, saying, "I'm no good." He needs frequent confirmation that he is good and that therapy will make him even better.

Whether treatment takes place in a busy clinic, at school, or in your very own basement, you will be involved, too. Part of the therapist's job is to collaborate with parents to design activities that help the child function better at home. The

The Out-of-Sync Child

therapist may also give suggestions to the teacher to modify the classroom environment.

Because treatment will become a part of your child's life, you and your child should get along well with the therapist. Goodness of fit is essential! If your child resists going for treatment, or if you lack confidence in the therapist, then something is amiss, and you should switch to another one, if possible. Treatment will be most successful when all the parties have a respectful and pleasant working relationship.

Working with the therapist will take some time and effort, but your involvement is definitely worthwhile. The therapy itself may not last forever, but the results will last a lifetime.

Keeping a Record

If you are not already keeping a running record of your child's behavior and development, please begin one now! Your record should include:

- Your own documented observations
- Teachers' comments and reports
- Names, addresses, and telephone numbers of professionals you have consulted or intend to consult
- Detailed, dated notes of consultations and telephone conversations with professionals
- Written confirmation of information you have received orally
- Specialists' evaluations, diagnoses, and recommendations

An orderly, chronological notebook is a valuable tool. It will help you see patterns that you may have missed. It will provide evidence of your child's uneven development, should you need to prove at some point that your child requires special services. It will also help you feel more organized and in control.

A professional diagnosis, along with therapy, should bring some relief. Meanwhile, life at home may improve when you follow some of the suggestions offered in the next chapter.

11

Your Child at Home

Parents can make home life easier both for themselves and their child by creating a sensory-enriched life, including activities that strengthen neurological development and improve self-help skills.

A Parent's Revelation

When Tonya was three, she entered St. Columba's. Reluctantly. She was fearful and limp. She spoke in a breathy voice, shrank from physical contact, and cried when it was time to go outdoors. However, she was very bright and loved stories, music, and dressing up.

During the fall, we screened the three-year-olds for SPD. Tonya's results suggested a possibility of some sensory processing differences, but we were not sure. She might have been simply immature.

While we usually observe late bloomers carefully before recommending occupational therapy, we decided to have a conference with Tonya's parents. We felt we could promote Tonya's social and physical development if we could persuade them to create a sensory-enriched life.

During the conference they listened politely to our

suggestions to get Tonya outside every day, to give her more hands-on experiences, and to invite children over to play.

"Well, those ideas won't work," her mother said. "Tonya hates being cold and messy. She dislikes going outside and playing with other kids. She just wants to be with the baby and me and listen to stories." Rising to her feet, she added, "And that's fine with us." Unsatisfactorily for all of us, the conference ended.

And so it went. Since the parents repeatedly resisted our suggestions, we decided to back off.

Then, just as we stepped back, Tonya's little sister took charge at home. This two-year-old began to clamor for changes in the family's lifestyle. Sociable and energetic, she loved playing outside with the neighborhood children. Her mother found that the best way to gratify her was to take her daily to the playground. Of course, Tonya had to go, too.

After the winter vacation, we noticed a "new" Tonya. She was participating more and playing happily with other children. She laughed, spoke up, and even shouted. Her development amazed and delighted us.

One day her mother said, "I must tell you, I've had a revelation. We've been going to the park every day, even when it is freezing. Tonya resisted at first, but now she asks to go. You had to tell me over and over again about offering more sensory-motor activities until I finally listened. Now I realize that for both girls, a sensory-enriched life makes good sense and a huge difference!"

A Sensory-Enriched Life

A "sensory-enriched life"—a term coined by Lindsey Biel, occupational therapist and coauthor of *Raising a Sensory Smart*

Child—is filled with fun and functional sensory-motor activities. An OT or other professional individualizes sensory experiences to meet the physical and emotional needs of a specific child's nervous system. The therapist suggests that parents weave these activities into the natural flow of home life to help the child become better regulated and more focused, adaptable, and skillful.

(A flexible, enjoyable program of family-centered activities differs from a "sensory diet." A sensory diet is a strict protocol that involves brushing the child's limbs with a specialized brush, compressing his joints in a very specific pattern, and putting fingers in his mouth for an oral swipe—every two hours.)

A sensory-enriched life includes a combination of alerting, organizing, and calming activities. An alerting or calming activity may come first, depending on your child's needs.

Alerting activities may especially benefit the sensory straggler, who needs a boost to become effectively aroused. These include:

- Crunching dry cereal, popcorn, chips, crackers, nuts, pretzels, carrots, celery, apples, or ice cubes,
- Taking a shower,
- Bouncing on a therapy ball or beach ball, or
- Jumping up and down on a mattress or trampoline.

Organizing activities help regulate the child's responses. They include:

- Chewing granola bars, fruit bars, licorice, dried apricots, cheese, gum, bagels, or bread crusts,

- Hanging by the hands from a chinning bar,
- Pushing or pulling heavy loads, or
- Getting into an upside-down position.

Calming activities help the child decrease sensory over-responsivity or overstimulation. They include:

- Sucking a pacifier, hard candy, frozen fruit bar, or spoonful of peanut butter,
- Pushing against walls with the hands, shoulders, back, buttocks, and head,
- Rocking, swaying, or swinging slowly to and fro,
- Cuddling or back rubbing, or
- Taking a bath.

When you initiate your own home program for a sensory-enriched life, it is always best to consult a therapist about your child's requirements. What are appropriate activities? Where should your child do them? When? How often? For how long?

Here are some guidelines:

- Set up specific times during the day for a structured sequence (after breakfast, after school, and before bedtime).
- If possible, supply the activity that your child wants. Often, the child will tell you. Even if he cannot say, "My nervous system desperately requires an intense move-ment experience," you may be able to read his mind as he prepares to leap from the porch roof. Find another way to let him jump!

- Let the child direct the play. While "More!" may mean more, do supervise so that the child does not become overaroused. "Stop!" means stop at once. During the activity, watch and listen for nonverbal signals: relaxation and pleased facial expressions suggest that the activity feels good; whimpers or raucous laughter suggest that it is time to cool down.
- For variety, change the routine and environment.
- Check periodically with the therapist to ensure that your home program is meeting your child's varying needs.

A sensory-enriched life is like a fitness plan. It will enhance every child's functioning, whether the child is in or out of sync.

Promoting Healthy Sensory Processing at Home

Many children seek more sensory experiences than others. They are touchers-and-feelers, bumpers-and-crashers. Their high activity level tells us that if they can play bumpety-bump on the tire swing, or soar into a leaf pile, or work with paint and clay, they will "get in sync." They are right.

Other children avoid sensory stimulation that makes them physically uncomfortable. Faced with the demand to touch or move around with certain objects, children with sensory issues may not know what they are supposed to do. Thus, they may seem uninterested in blocks, balls, bread dough, or bicycles. The result is that they get stuck, and the less they do, the less they can do.

What helps? Practice, practice, practice! These children need guidance to explore their environment and to feel safe. Once they learn how to play actively, they begin to get in sync.

Also, they need objects with plenty of affordances. The term "affordance," coined by the psychologist James J. Gibson,[1] describes something about an object in the environment that invites a person's interaction.

Consider the cardboard tube. Occupational therapists Teresa May-Benson, ScD, and Sharon Cermak, EdD, have researched how children with different sensory processing abilities respond when handed a tube and told, "Show me what you can do with this."[2] Most kids will quickly demonstrate how you can see, listen, blow, or sing through it. You can drop marbles into it. You can strike your knee with it. It is rollable, tossable, catchable, stick-your-fingers-into-able. (An affordance, you will note, ends with the suffix "-able," including "affordable"!)

Children with SPD, however, demonstrate fewer affordances when handed a cardboard tube. Dr. Ayres found that children with dyspraxia interact ineffectively with objects in their environment because it is hard for them to ideate what to do, plan how to do it, and execute their plan.[3]

Following are some ideas for multisensory activities to help children get in sync. Simple equipment, known as "beautiful junk" and found around the house, includes straws, paper plates, buttons, and masking tape.

Every child can benefit from these suggestions—not just children who seek such activities, but also more tentative children, as well as siblings and friends.

Want more? For hundreds of detailed activities for children of all ages, see About the Author (page 381) for information about my book *The Out-of-Sync Child Has Fun*, and other publications coauthored with Joye Newman: *Growing an In-Sync Child*, *In-Sync Activity Cards*, *A Year of Mini-Moves for the In-Sync Child*, and the In-Sync Child Method webinars.

ACTIVITIES TO DEVELOP THE TACTILE SYSTEM

Tactile Road—Provide various surfaces for your child to move across, such as grass, sand, carpet, velvet, satin, bubble wrap, fake fur, corrugated cardboard, sandpaper, and a cabdriver's wooden-bead car-seat cover. Barefoot is best, and even with shoes on, the child will get valuable input.

Back Drawing—With your finger, "draw" a shape, letter, number, or design on the child's back or hand. Ask the child to guess what it is and then draw the design on another person's back.

Treasure Trove—Put sand, beans, rice, pasta, or mud in a plastic tub. Add small cars, people, and animals for the child to arrange, bury, and rediscover. If getting messy is too challenging, offer vinyl gloves.

People Sandwich—Have the "salami" or "turkey" (your child) lie facedown on the "bread" (gym mat or couch). With a "spreader" (your hands, or a sponge, vegetable brush, or washcloth), smear her limbs and torso with pretend mustard, mayonnaise, relish, etc. Use firm, downward strokes. Cover the child from her neck down with another piece of "bread" (folded mat or couch cushions). Now press firmly on the mat to squish out the excess mustard and to provide deep, soothing pressure.

Time Inn—Find space in your home or yard for a cozy getaway for your child. Unlike a punitive time-out place, this is a restorative asylum where a child can calm down and be comfortable. It could be a refrigerator carton, beanbag chair, hammock, teepee, or "fort" under the dining room table.

ACTIVITIES TO DEVELOP THE VESTIBULAR SYSTEM

Balancing on a Teeter-Totter—Center a board over a wooden timber. Your child can walk, jump, or crawl from one end of the board to the other, sit or stand over the fulcrum and tip from side to side, and pull or push the board back onto the timber after it slips off.

Teeter-Totter:

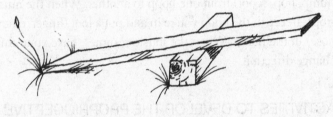

Sitting on a T-Stool—The wiggliest child will find her center on a T-stool when she discovers the tripod formula (her two feet in front and the stool leg directly underneath). To make one, connect two 12-inch sections of a two-by-four with two long wood screws. Sitting on a T-stool is guaranteed to improve balance, posture, and—amazingly so—attention.

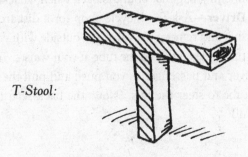

T-Stool:

Rocking Boat—Have your child lie on her stomach, grab her ankles behind her, and rock to and fro. This develops not only the vestibular system but also proprioception, motor planning, and much more.

Rolling Log—Scatter a few beanbags around the floor. Say to your child, "Stretch out on the floor as straight as a log. Look at the red beanbag and roll to it. Put your head on it. Now roll to the blue beanbag."

Stop-and-Go Hoops—Scatter hoops or paper plates around. Say, "When I start the music, show me how you walk (jump, hop, scoot) from one hoop to another. When the music stops, freeze in the hoop you're in and put a foot (finger, elbow, nose) in the hoop." When the music resumes, have your child change direction.

ACTIVITIES TO DEVELOP THE PROPRIOCEPTIVE SYSTEM

Paper Bag Kickball—Kicking and hitting are good survival skills to have. Instead of you or other living things being the punching bag, provide a paper grocery bag for your angry or frustrated child. Open the bag fully. Scrunch the opening closed to make it ball-like. Alone or with a group, the child can kick and punch the bag with gusto. An alternative is a standing, inflatable punching bag that bounces back when whacked.

Bus Driver—Ask the bicycle shop for a discarded inner tube. Wash it and remove the valve. Go outside with your child, step into the circle, and hold the tube at your waists. Take turns being driver and passenger as you push and pull the resistive, stretchy tube to steer the bus. (Note: the back-seat driver has all the fun!)

Amazing Delivery Kid—Have the child lift and carry grocery bags, filled with potato sacks, soda bottles, and other non-breakables, into the house. Have him haul the laundry basket upstairs or lug a box of books, a bucket of blocks, or a pail of water from one spot to another.

More Core—Sit beside your child against a wall, legs straight out. Press your back and shoulders to the wall. Say, "Let's stretch so that we are sitting very tall and pushing back so that there's hardly any space between our backs and the wall. Now let's slide our arms along the wall, up over our heads. Now let's lower our arms slowly to the floor." Repeat.

ACTIVITIES TO DEVELOP THE AUDITORY SYSTEM

Tapping Tunes—Tap or clap the rhythm of a familiar song, such as "Jingle Bells" or "Row, Row, Row Your Boat." Ask your child to guess the tune. Hum it or sing a few key words to make the game easier. Take turns.

Keyboard Tales—Sit at a piano keyboard together and tell the story of "Goldilocks," "Three Little Pigs," or another tale with three to five characters. Strike a few bass notes and say in a low voice, "Papa Bear sounds like this." Play an octave higher for Mama Bear, another octave higher for Goldilocks, and a few treble notes for Baby Bear. Tell the story while your child bangs out notes in the appropriate range and speaks the characters' lines.

Zop and Hop—Say, "I'll say a nonsense word, 'zop.' 'Zop' rhymes with another word that means a way of moving. Yes, it's 'hop'!" Have your child rhyme and demonstrate more movements using nonsense words such as "brump" (jump), "garch" (march), and "bipboe" (tiptoe).

Rubber Band Harp—Provide an open wooden box (like a cigar box, with the lid removed) and rubber bands. Your child can choose bands to stretch over the box and then strum or pluck the "harp strings" to accompany favorite songs. Many children with SPD and autism have excellent musical pitch, so "tuning" the harp may be fun. To make a plucked rubber band sound higher, pull it behind the box so it tightens in front. To make it lower, pull it toward the front to loosen it. You can feel, hear, and see how the bands behave differently, depending on their tension.

ACTIVITIES TO DEVELOP THE VISUAL SYSTEM

Guesstimation—Gather two spaghetti boxes and various small items, such as paper clips, toothpicks, buttons, and Legos. Place the boxes side by side, six inches apart. Ask, "How many paper clips do you think could line up between the boxes?"

How Many Steps?—This is another estimating game to develop spatial awareness and other visual skills. Ask, "How many steps (jumps, stomps, hops) will it take to walk from the door to the sink?"

Napkin Origami—On a piece of paper, draw a rectangle, square, and triangle. Hand your child a napkin. Point to the rectangle and say, "Fold the napkin to make it look like this shape." Continue. Have him place a folded napkin beside each plate at the table.

Wall Ball—On a wall, stick a horizontal line of masking tape at your child's shoulder height. Hand him a ball and say, "Show me how you can roll this ball along the tape to the end, using your hands." Make this eye-tracking activity harder by taping vertical, zigzag, or curvy lines.

MORE ACTIVITIES TO DEVELOP SENSORY-MOTOR SKILLS

Sensory processing is the foundation for fine-motor skills, oral-motor skills, motor planning, and bilateral coordination. All these skills improve as the child tries the following activities that integrate the sensations.

Fine-Motor Skills

Toothpick Constructions—Let your child stick toothpicks into food chunks such as cucumbers, beans, popcorn, fruit, cheese, firm tofu, or marshmallows. She can construct houses, robots, porcupines, and other creations, and then eat them up.

Make-a-Ball—Provide rubber bands for your child to stretch over a ping-pong ball.

Paper Clip Designs—Place several paper clips on one edge of a notecard. Say, "Can you put paper clips on your card so that they look like my pattern?" Take turns designing and copying more complex designs.

Sticky Bracelet—On your child's wrist, wrap a "bracelet" of masking tape, not too tight, sticky side out. Provide buttons, sequins, alphabet noodles, paper scraps, and other small items to make a lovely bracelet.

Oral-Motor Skills

Applesauce Through a Straw—Offer pureed applesauce, pudding, or a frozen fruit drink for your child to suck up through a short, thick straw.

Spirited Shepherds—Gather cotton balls (sheep), markers, straws, and a pie pan (corral). "Brand" everyone's cotton balls with a distinct color. Say, "Let's herd our sheep toward the corral." Get on the floor and "herd" your sheep by blowing them toward the corral. Once there, suck in through the straw to airlift the sheep and release them safely into the corral.

Bubble Gum—the bigger the wad, the better! Chewing gum and making bubbles is excellent therapy and provides oral satisfaction. Kids' "chewies" (available on the Internet) are good alternatives when gum is not an option.

Motor Planning

Paper Plate Affordances—To interact effectively with their environment, children with SPD need extra time to practice toying with objects. Provide a paper plate and say, "Show me what you can do." A plate is rollable, foldable, ripable, tossable, write-on-able, and skate-on-able. What other affordances can your child ideate, make a motor plan for, and then perform?

Jumpland—Have your child stand on a low step. Ask, "How far can you jump?" After each landing, mark the spot with chalk. Encourage him to jump farther each time.

Push-Me-Pull-You—Load a wagon with beanbags or bags of rice. Have your child push or pull the wagon between and around obstacles (traffic cones, wastebaskets, etc.) placed about five feet apart.

Nose to Knee—Say, "Get on your hands and knees and make your body look like a table. Now round your back and bring your nose and knee together. Straighten that leg, keep your knee off the floor, and look at the sky. Now be flat as a table again." Repeat on other side.

Bilateral Coordination

Marble Trails—Line a tray with paper. Put a few dabs of finger paint in the center of the paper. Provide a marble to roll through the paint to make a design. Great wrapping paper!

Arm Circles—Say, "Extend your arms to the sides and rotate them in small circles ten times. Now reverse direction. Now overhead. Now behind you."

Clap Your Feet—Say, "Show me how you clap your hands, nod your head, shake your head, scrunch your face, wiggle your thumbs, and roll your hands. Great! Can you also clap your feet, nod your pointer fingers, shake your hands, scrunch your hands and feet, wiggle your big toes, and roll your feet?"

Stretch Like Me—Play this follow-the-leader game with three or more people. Everyone needs a yard-long stretchy exercise band. Say, "Watch and follow my move." Count to eight as you demonstrate your move eight times. Say, "Let's do it together." Then say, "Now it is your turn. Stretch your band your own way, and everyone will follow you." Give everyone a turn to be the leader.

SUGGESTIONS TO DEVELOP SELF-HELP SKILLS

Self-help skills improve along with sensory processing. The following suggestions may make your child's life easier—and yours, too!

Dressing

Let your child choose what to wear. If she gets overheated easily, let her go outdoors wearing several loose layers rather than a coat. If she complains that new clothes are stiff or scratchy, let her wear soft, worn clothes, even if they're unfashionable. Comfort is what matters.

In your child's bureau and closet, eliminate unnecessary choices, such as clothes that are outgrown or inappropriate for the season.

Put large hooks inside closet doors at the child's eye level so he can hang up his coat and pajamas.

Supply cellophane bags for the child to slip her feet into before pulling on boots. The cellophane prevents shoes from getting stuck and makes the job much easier.

Snack and Meal Time

Provide a chair, therapy ball, or T-stool that allows the child's elbows to be at table height and feet to be flat on the floor. (A stool or pillow may help the fidgety kid to feel grounded.)

Offer a variety of foods with different textures: lumpy, smooth, crunchy, chewy. Keep portions small, especially when introducing new foods.

Let the child pour juice or milk into a cup. The child who frequently overreaches or spills juice needs much practice. A tipless cup will help prevent accidents.

Encourage the child to handle snack-time or mealtime objects. Opening cracker packages, spreading peanut butter, and eating with utensils are good for proprioception, bilateral coordination, and fine-motor skills.

Chores

Together, make a list of chores he can do to help around the house: Make his bed, walk the dog, empty wastebaskets, take out trash, pull weeds, rake, shovel, sweep, vacuum, fold laundry, empty the dishwasher, set and clear the table. Let him know you need and appreciate him.

Stick to a routine. When he finishes a chore, let him put a star on the chart. Reward him with a special privilege or outing when he accumulates several stars. Divide chores into small steps. Let him clear the table one plate at a time. (He doesn't have to clear all the dishes.)

Bathing

Let the child help regulate the water temperature. She may like it hotter or cooler than you do. Offer an assortment of bath toys, soaps, and scrubbers. Provide a large bath sheet, warmed in the dryer, for a tight wrap-up.

Sleeping

Give notice: "Half an hour until bedtime!" or "You can draw for five more minutes."

Stick to a bedtime routine. Include stories and songs, a look at a sticker collection, a chat about today's events or tomorrow's plans, a back rub, and a snug tuck-in.

For tactilely overresponsive children, provide comfortable pajamas. Some like them loose, some like them tight; some like them silky, some do not like them at all. Nobody likes them bumpy, scratchy, lacy, or with elasticized cuffs.

Use percale or silk sheets for a smooth and bumpless bed.

Let your child sleep with extra pillows and blankets, in a sleeping bag or bed tent, or on a waterbed.

Life at home can improve with a sensory-enriched life and attention to your child's special needs, and life at school can improve as well.

12

Your Child at School

Becoming an advocate for your child, communicating with school personnel, finding a good school-and-child match, and sharing ideas with teachers can all promote your child's success at school.

What a Difference Communication Makes!

Last year, Nicky hated fourth grade. Mrs. Colladay, his teacher, was mean. She always scolded him when he was slow, disorganized, or fidgety. She would say, "I wish you would just try harder." He was trying.

This year, Nicky loves fifth grade. Ms. Berry is nice. She makes sure he understands the assignments and shows him how to break them down into manageable parts. She got him a chair that does not wiggle and thick pencils that do not break. She made him captain of the Flying Aces Math Team. She never makes him miss recess. She likes him.

What a difference a teacher makes! And what a difference a parent makes when she becomes her child's advocate!

Nicky is in a classroom that meets his needs because his mother took action. After years of seeking to avoid stigma and labels, she decided to inform the school about his sensory processing problems and about the benefits of therapy and a sensory-enriched life. If Nicky could function more smoothly at home, surely he could gain confidence and competence at school.

During the summer, Nicky's mother met with the principal and Ms. Berry and was relieved to find them eager for information. They wanted to understand Nicky's strengths and weaknesses so they could promote his success. They told her they would explain his needs to the art, science, and physical education teachers. They would arrange for special services at school. They would call her with questions and would welcome her calls.

What a difference communication makes!

If Only School Were More Like Home

The child with SPD often has enormous difficulty in the classroom. His problem is not a lack of intelligence or willingness to learn. His problem may be dyspraxia, which is difficulty in knowing what to do and how to go about doing it.

The preschooler who has difficulty stringing beads often becomes the school-age child who cannot organize the parts of a research project. He wants to interact successfully with the world around him, but he cannot easily adapt his behavior to meet increasingly complex demands.

The out-of-sync child may be unable to settle down to work. Everything may be distracting—the proximity of a classmate, the sound of rustling paper, the movement of children playing outside the window, the scratchy label inside his shirt collar, and even the tippy chairs and tables. He may be disorganized in his movements, verbal responses, and interactions with teachers and classmates.

For many reasons, school may be grueling:

1) School puts pressure on children to perform and conform. While the average child buckles down to meet expectations, the out-of-sync child buckles under pressure.

2) The school milieu is ever-changing. Abrupt transitions from circle time to art projects, from math to reading, or from cafeteria to gymnasium may overwhelm the child who switches gears slowly.

3) Sensory stimuli may be excessive. People mill around. Lights, sounds, and odors abound. The child may become overloaded easily.

4) Sensory stimuli may be insufficient. A long stretch of sitting may pose problems for the child who regularly needs short stretching breaks to organize his body. A spoken or written lesson, directed toward aural and visual learners, may not reach the kinesthetic and tactile learner.

5) School administrators and teachers often misunderstand SPD. They may be truly interested in helping the child, but they cannot accommodate his unique learning style if they do not know where to begin.

6) School is not like home. For many children, school is unpredictable and risky, while home is familiar and safe. (On the other hand, sometimes school is orderly and predictable, while home is stressful and chaotic.) The behavior of the child will differ because the environments differ. School can become more like home, however, when parents share information about their child with the adults who can make a difference in the child's success.

Years ago, before we became savvy about sensory processing, the St. Columba's director and I met with Allen's mother to
learn how we could support her boy. At preschool, he hardly
spoke, hardly moved. He would park himself in the sandbox
corner, behind a barricade of trucks. He had no self-help skills,
no playmates, no affect. We described a sad, scared, helpless
loner.

His mother was astonished. "But he is not that way at all!"
she said. Her description was 180 degrees different from ours.
At home, he was a chatterbox. He was lively and cheerful.
He jumped on the furniture, dug in the garden, and played
with neighborhood kids. True, the kids he played with were
all younger. True, he had trouble getting dressed. True, he had
definite likes and dislikes in foods and activities. But he was
not a problem at home. "If only school were more like home,"
she said with a sigh.

The conference was an eye-opener for everyone. As we
talked, his mother realized that Allen functioned well at home
because she fulfilled his need for consistent routines, just-right
stimulation, physical security, and constant reminders of love.
We, the teachers, realized that we could fulfill some of those
needs at school, now that we understood what they were.

We entered a home-and-school partnership to help Allen
succeed. The teachers became more sensitive to his cautious
behavior and learned to guide him gently into preschool activities. They gave him more structure and protected him from
overstimulation. Many small changes had a big, positive effect
on his behavior.

Meanwhile, his mother adapted Allen's home environment
to meet his special needs. She found room in the house for a
trampoline, crawling tunnel, therapy ball, gym mat, beanbag
chair, and indoor swing, so Allen could get a great sensory-motor

"workout" in the morning before school. She also became aware of her obligation to share her observations, selectively, with his school and teachers.

Deciding Whom to Tell

The out-of-sync child needs an articulate advocate. Usually, it is up to a parent to make teachers and other caregivers aware of the child's special needs.

The thought of revealing their child's difficulties makes many parents anxious. They worry that the child may be stigmatized and labeled, that they may be blamed for the child's behavior, or that insensitive school personnel may be indiscreet or may use the information in the wrong way. Besides, talking about the child's inadequacies is painful. Nonetheless, for the child's sake, communication is essential.

Why is it necessary to provide information? Adults who work with children, like sculptors who work with clay, must have a feel for the material they shape. With some understanding of SPD, they can become more attuned to the child's differing abilities. Without information, however, they cannot be expected to change their classroom environment, alter their teaching style, or redirect their thinking.

Who needs to know? Classroom teachers should be informed. The principal; the art, science, music, and physical education teachers; and the computer and media specialists may need to know. School bus and carpool drivers, religious-school teachers, scout leaders, coaches, and babysitters also may be more considerate when told.

What information should be shared? Briefly, tell the teacher what the child's problem is. (Avoid terms such as "underresponsivity to vestibular sensations," unless pressed for details.) Then give specific suggestions about what works at home so the teacher can consider doing the same at school.

Examples: "My daughter is very sensitive to being touched or jostled. At home, we have noticed she does best when she doesn't feel crowded. Would you remember her need for space when you plan the seating arrangement?" Or, "My son has difficulty with motor coordination. He is receiving therapy to help him move more smoothly. At home, we find that frequent breaks to move and stretch help him get organized."

When you find that the teacher is receptive, you may also choose to share your own documented observations, therapists' evaluations, sensory-enriched life suggestions, and tips for teachers, included at the end of this chapter.

How should information be shared? Frame the information positively: "She concentrates beautifully if . . ." or "His motor coordination improves when . . ." Stress the child's abilities: "She adores art projects" or "He has a great sense of humor." Enlist the teacher's goodwill: "We hope we can work together. Please keep me posted!"

Where should information be shared? Arrange meetings in advance so that you and the teacher can talk uninterrupted. Confer in the classroom before or after school, in the teachers' lounge at lunchtime, or by telephone at night.

When should information be shared? Before the school year starts, anticipate your child's difficulties and communicate with those who need to know. Help them be proactive, rather than reactive, when problems arise.

A Good School-and-Child Match

Communicating regularly with school personnel should make a positive difference for your child. Sometimes, however, the teacher will resist taking suggestions and making accommodations, even if your child is legally entitled to them. You will then have to decide whether to step in or step back.

For instance, one mother knew that chewing gum helped her son get organized while reading and writing. She asked the teacher if gum would be permissible. The teacher refused: "He cannot have special privileges just because he has special needs." Although the mother was reluctant to go over the teacher's head and make a fuss, she decided to complain to the principal. The principal intervened, the teacher relented, and the child was allowed to chew (but not crack) gum. His performance improved, and several months later, the teacher apologized.

Sometimes, the teacher is willing to make adjustments, but the school resists. The child may benefit from a therapy ball seat instead of a chair, or a desk of his own rather than a shared table, or a locker he can open easily, while the school insists on regulation furnishings. In such cases, pick the most important battles—and keep fighting.

If goodness-of-fit at school is lacking, you have several options:

- Ask to move the child to another teacher's classroom.
- Investigate special-education programs. Special-education classes are smaller and less distracting than regular classrooms. Special educators are trained to address children's differing abilities. With an IEP, the out-of-sync child may flourish.
- Transfer the child from one public school to another. An advantage of public education is the availability of facilities, including OTs, speech therapists, and remedial reading specialists. If the child is eligible for special

education, these services are provided during the school day, at no charge.

- Enroll the child in a private school, with smaller class size and more individualized attention. In a private school the immature child can repeat a grade, if necessary, whereas in a public school the child may not get this chance to "pause" before promotion to a more challenging grade.

- Homeschool your child. Many children learn best at home, where they can go at their own pace without distractions. Participating in after-school activities is still your child's right and is also a good idea to encourage social interactions with other children.

Each school year, reopen the channels of communication. Teachers will come and go—some sensitive, some not so sensitive—and your steady support and voice will help your child succeed.

Below you will find some classroom strategies to share with your child's teacher. He or she may learn from these guidelines how to be supportive; how to gauge when to encourage and when to step back; how to refrain from overloading the child with excessive stimulation and unmanageable work; and how to control his or her own frustrations when dealing with an out-of-sync child.

Promoting Your Child's Success at School

The child with SPD needs understanding and support if he is going to succeed at school, whether that school is public or private. A teacher may want to help an out-of-sync student but may lack training in the appropriate techniques. If so, the teacher may wish to try some of the following classroom strategies that will help the out-of-sync child. They will also help every other child.

Yes, every child!

Every child benefits from a safe, calm, and distraction-free environment. Every child requires frequent breaks from work to move and stretch. Every child needs to know that someone is paying attention to his strengths and weaknesses, likes and dislikes, ups and downs. Every child needs to be shown how to find solutions to problems. Every child needs assurance that it's okay to have differing abilities, that he can be successful, that his ideas have merit, that his personhood is valued.

When the out-of-sync child begins to feel more in control, his schoolwork and social skills will improve. When he is less distracted, he distracts the other children less. Then, when all the students are working to the best of their ability, the teacher can teach!

CLASSROOM STRATEGIES

Controlling the Environment

Reduce sensory overload. You may have to intuit what kind of sensory stimulation is getting in the child's way because he may be unable to tell you. Remember that stimuli that bother him today may not bother him tomorrow, and vice versa. If you can remove or diminish most distractions, you will increase the child's ability to attend to the important job of learning. Help the child focus on one idea at a time by minimizing unrelated sensory stimuli. Simplify, simplify, simplify.

Tactile distractions may divert the child's attention. If the proximity of classmates irritates the child, help him find a spot where he will feel safe. Steer the preschooler to a seat at the head of the table, or at the edge of the rug, to lessen the possibility of contact with other children. Station the elementary school child's desk in a classroom corner or up front near you.

Let her bring up the rear when the class tiptoes single file down the corridor so that no one can bump her from behind. Provide her with the space she needs.

Visual distractions may interfere with the child's concentration. Eliminate clutter on bulletin boards. Secure artwork, maps, and graphics on the walls so that they do not flutter. Tack a sheet over open shelves to cover art materials, games, and toys that may attract the child's attention. Remove mobiles swaying from light fixtures. Adjust window blinds to prevent sunshine from flickering through.

The movements of other children may also be visually distracting. Have the child sit near you at the front of the room, with his back to his classmates. Surround him with children who sit quietly, pay attention, and serve as good role models.

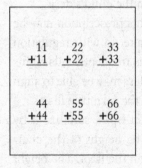
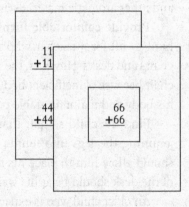

When preparing worksheets for the school-age child, keep to a minimum the instructions to read and math problems to solve. White space around each written problem helps the child focus on one at a time. He may do best when he can frame each problem with a cardboard template.

Auditory distractions may make the room seem like an echo chamber for the child with auditory processing differences. A classroom's hard surfaces, such as desktops, linoleum tiles, and painted walls, reflect sound. Wherever possible, cover hard surfaces with carpet, cloth, or corkboard. Be sure the child is not seated near the humming fish tank, under the buzzing fluorescent bulb, or beside the window, where he may be distracted by children's voices outside.

When the children are working at their desks, you may find that playing classical music, such as Bach and Mozart, softens the auditory environment and helps organize everybody.

Olfactory distractions may include the smells coming from the lunchroom or from the gerbil cage. If it is possible to adjust the schedule, time your lessons so that the child's most difficult subject is not being taught as the fragrance of grilled cheese wafts through the door. Keep animals, paint supplies, and other aromatic materials away from the child's desk.

Provide comfortable furniture. This prescription may be hard to fill for a teacher who must make do with regulation chairs and desks. However, the child who frequently falls off his chair because of inefficient body awareness may be able to align his body and maintain stable posture if the furniture fits.

Find the child a chair that does not tip or stabilize it by jamming the legs into tennis balls. The height of the chair should allow him to place his feet flat on the floor. The height of the desk should be at his waist level.

An older child who is expected to sit at a desk for long periods might benefit from a textured cushion that will help him stick to the seat. (A teenage boy, whose sensory problems had been overlooked for years, glued thumbtacks—points UP—to the seat of his desk chair at home. The tacks, he explained, reminded him when he was about to slide off the chair! A cushion would seem to be a preferable alternative.) If the other students want to try the cushion, let them. Soon they will forget about it, and you can get on with your job while the child who needs it stays put.

Sometimes, a special type of chair helps. If the child is fidgety at his seat, for instance, a ball to sit on will help focus his attention. The ball's diameter should equal the distance between his buttocks and the floor when his knees are bent at a right angle and his feet are flat on the floor.

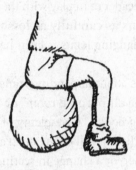

Staying put in a designated spot on the floor is easy for the younger child when he is seated in a HowdaHUG, a slatted, wooden "sensory chair." Like a stadium or camping seat, this item provides postural support and improves attention while allowing the child to rock and wiggle. See www.howda.com.

Keep boards and worksheets clean. Fuzzy lines present problems for the child with visual processing difficulties. Most helpful are crisp white lines on a dark chalkboard and clear dark lines on white paper so that the child can discriminate between the background and the letters or numbers you want her to understand.

Managing the Classroom

Develop a consistent routine. The out-of-sync child may have trouble getting organized to do what is necessary. He may struggle to overcome a feeling of chaos, internally and externally. Thus, he is most comfortable when things are "just so," exactly as they were yesterday and will be tomorrow. His rigidity is a manifestation of his need to organize his world.

For this child, a classroom that is clearly structured is preferable to one that runs on spontaneity. Help him by writing classroom routines on the board, sticking to the schedule, keeping the room arranged in a predictable way, and remembering whose turn it is to be line leader or to play with the new set of magnets.

Plan transitions as carefully as lessons. If focusing on a task is difficult, changing focus is even harder for the out-of-sync child.

Notify students about impending transitions: "In ten minutes, we'll go to the all-purpose room" or "After recess, you'll get the new reading books." Give plenty of notice when something out of the ordinary will occur, such as a field trip, a visit from a reptile trainer, or a change in seating arrangements.

To facilitate transitions, signify what will happen next by clapping or beating drum rhythms. For instance, two long claps followed by three short claps may say that it is time to put away math books and stand up to stretch.

$$\overline{\text{long}}, \overline{\text{long}}, \text{short}, \text{short}, \overline{\text{short}}$$

A sequence of one long clap followed by four short claps and a final long clap may mean that it is time to come in from the schoolyard.

$$\overline{\text{long}}, \overline{\text{short}}, \overline{\text{short}}, \overline{\text{short}}, \overline{\text{short}}, \overline{\text{long}}$$

Prepare transition fillers to turn empty time into teachable moments. Recite poems and sing activity songs with motions. Offer activities to strengthen language and critical-thinking skills, such as passing around laminated "What's missing?" pages from children's magazines, or playing "What if?" games (What if we had wings? What if we had no electricity?).

Brainstorm together. Write down everyone's suggestions for class plays or for science projects. Assure each child that his idea is valid.

Take a vote. Who wants a happy face on the jack-o'-lantern and who wants a scary face? Who hopes the Democrat will win and who chooses the Republican? Who wants to study rain forests and who prefers deserts?

Plan movement breaks between and during activities. Provide acceptable ways for the fidgety child to move. Incorporate movement into the routine so children can stand and stretch, or move across the room from math to the science center, or march to a drumbeat. Try activities such as Simon Says (where nobody loses), follow-the-leader, jumping jacks, or relay races. Play silent speedball, in which the children pass a ball quickly around a circle without making a peep. Movement stimulates the brain and body and helps every child pay attention, think, speak, and write.

Devise team or club efforts. Teams that read the most books, solve the most math problems, or produce cooperative projects earn a reward that you can decide on together. Earning team points can be a strong incentive for out-of-sync students as well as for better-organized classmates who may not choose to work with them.

Helping Children Become Better Organized

Encourage students to be active rather than passive learners. All children have an inner drive to learn, and they learn best when they can move and touch. Remember that reading and listening are not every child's main avenue of learning. Therefore, provide multisensory lessons so that the learning arrives through every possible route.

For example, the preschooler with inefficient auditory processing may learn best through tactile and visual experiences. Thus, he may learn more about rhythm and pitch by playing "Jingle Bells" on the xylophone than by hearing a recording. The older child whose visual processing problem makes worksheets a chore may learn well in hands-on, real-life situations. Thus, he can absorb math concepts while making change in a school store.

Many children with SPD have narrow interests. Find out what the child has an affinity for and lead her to explore the subject she is passionate about through her preferred sensory path. Is she interested in spiders? Planets? Native Americans? If she is a tactile learner, let her draw a picture or build a model. If she likes to talk, let her give a short oral presentation. If she loves to move, let her demonstrate ritual dances. Build on the child's sensory strengths. Then give her books to read in the area in which she has expertise. Even prereaders learn best when they can investigate subjects that they consider interesting and relevant.

Post this Chinese proverb in your classroom as a constant reminder:

I hear, and I forget.
I see, and I remember.
I do, and I understand.

Give children time. Nobody likes to feel rushed, especially the child with SPD, who may take longer than others to process new information. This child needs warm-up time just as much as cool-down time.

Give this child the luxury of time to learn new material:

A) Before presenting a lesson, tell the class what you will teach them,
B) Teach them,
C) Tell them what you have taught them, and then
D) Allow them time to absorb the lesson or to practice it. Drill is particularly valuable for the child who, lacking an internal sense of order, requires repetition of academic tasks before catching on.

Give the child time to process a question and answer. The special child often has the knowledge but just takes longer to prove it. Ten seconds is not too long to wait for an answer that someone else may produce in three.

Simplify instructions. When you give instructions, make eye contact with the child if possible. (Children with SPD or autism frequently are uncomfortable with eye contact and can listen better when they are not forced to look you in the eye.) Give one or two directions at a time. Be concise and specific. Repeat the instructions if necessary. When assigning daily homework, say it in words and put it in writing. Have the child repeat it and write it down herself.

Short assignments will match the child's short attention span, will help him see an end to the task, and will give him a series of little successes.

Break down big assignments into small chunks. He may be a great reader but have difficulty planning long-term research projects. Provide a schedule and your clear expectations. For example, Week 1: Each child will tell you his chosen topic.

Week 2: He will submit a tentative reading list. Week 3: An outline. Week 4: A rough draft. Week 5: A finished report.

Provide a choice of writing implements. Some children do better with standard pencils, others with fat primary pencils; some with standard crayons, others with chubby crayons. While fine-motor skills generally develop later in boys than in girls, these skills are especially late-blooming in the boy or girl with SPD. Help the child choose the writing tool that fits him or her best.

Respect the child's needs. The child's primary need is to feel safe. When he feels safe, his brain is available for learning.

Many fine teachers, with the best intentions, commonly err with children by trying to jolly them out of their sensory issues. For instance, a teacher may tell the preschooler with tactile overresponsivity that "everyone likes finger paint, so take your turn," hoping to change his tendency to withdraw from touch. A physical education teacher of the older child with vestibular overresponsivity may try to position him to do a somersault on the tumbling mat. These encouragements won't "fix" the child's difficulty but instead may cause an aversive response, because he feels threatened.

Unless you know exactly what you're doing, it is better to respect the child's sensory differences. Remember that the child's behavior is out of line not because he won't do things right but because he can't. It is unfair to force the child to do things he is not ready to do.

Give the child alternatives. Anticipate problems and help the child find suitable alternatives to situations that cause the problems. For example, the child who is uncoordinated may avoid boisterous recess games. Guide him to other activities he can excel in that will strengthen his motor skills and that won't make him feel like a bystander or a baby.

For the preschooler, the opportunity to go through an obstacle course at his own pace, after everyone else has completed it, is one possibility. If he resists a particular obstacle, such as the balance beam or tunnel, let him be! Praise him for conquering the obstacles he can manage.

For the older child, ball skills may improve after playing tetherball, one-on-one catching and throwing games, or dribbling activities with a teacher or a buddy.

In the classroom, the child who is easily distracted by too many choices may seem unable to choose any. He may say he's bored when he is really confused. Help him find an activity or project that he can do while socializing with just one or two other children.

If possible, consult with an occupational therapist about classroom modifications, educationally relevant activities, and sensory-motor techniques you can use to address the child's special needs during the school day.

Adapting Your Own Behavior

Emphasize the positive. Give each child what psychotherapist Carl R. Rogers calls "unconditional, positive regard." The child with SPD needs constant assurance that her efforts are appreciated and worthwhile. She may not feel competent even when she is! Reward the child for what she did accomplish rather than remarking about what she left undone. Success breeds success.

Keep your voice low. The child with a supersensitive auditory system can become very uncomfortable when he hears a high-pitched or loud voice. He may even misinterpret your tone of voice and become distraught.

One day, I had to use a more forceful voice than usual to move a group of preschoolers through a Halloween song in which different rhythm instruments represented witches, skeletons, and pumpkins. Midway through the song, I raised my voice to be heard: "Now, please put down your tambourines and pick up your wood blocks."

I did not understand then, although I do now, why a particularly anxious boy cried, "Don't talk to me that way! Don't you know I can't do anything right when you talk to me that way?" My words had not been threatening; my directions had not been complicated. It was my louder, higher voice that made him fall apart. More effective would have been whispering, the technique I learned to use, especially in a noisy room.

Provide physical feedback. When you want to be certain that the child is paying attention, get up close. Look the child in the eye, if that does not make the child uncomfortable. While speaking, put your hands on the child's shoulders and press down firmly. These techniques may help the child focus better on what you are saying.

Keep your expectations realistic. So what if the child does not complete a task or does it differently from the way other children do it? Remember what is most important in learning: process rather than product, and participation rather than perfection.

13

Coping with Your
Child's Emotions

For the child to become more self-regulated and for families to deal with the emotional fallout of SPD, there are positive words and actions that may improve the child's skills and self-esteem, as well as pitfalls to avoid.

A Typically Dreadful Morning

Marge, the mother of two, tells this story:

> This morning was typically dreadful. Chip, my eight-year-old, got out of bed on the wrong side. Actually, he fell out of bed. Then, on his way to the bathroom, he crashed into Melissa and knocked her down. He yelled at her, "You're always in my way, dumb head!" She ran downstairs, bawling. He's always so mean to her, and she's only three.
>
> While I comforted her, I heard Chip slamming his bureau drawers and shouting. He finally came downstairs wearing his T-shirt inside out. He said this way the tags wouldn't hurt him. I thought that was pretty good

problem-solving, but my husband disagreed. Before I could say anything, he ordered Chip to change. Chip refused. My husband was furious. He pulled off Chip's shirt, turned it right side out, and stuffed Chip into it. Chip was really upset and fighting back tears.

Finally, he sat down and poured orange juice over his cereal. When I said that wasn't a good idea, he began to cry. He said, "It was an accident! I didn't do it on purpose!" Then he poured the rest of the juice on Melissa's head. On purpose.

Okay. I kept my temper, because it was time to meet the school bus. But Chip couldn't find his reading book. It took ten minutes to find it behind the couch. He missed the bus, so I drove him to school. When we got there, we saw a classmate getting out of her car. She had a model of an igloo made of sugar cubes. Then Chip really lost control. He had forgotten about the "homes around the world" assignment. I felt just awful because I had forgotten, too. Chip hunkered down and refused to get out of the car.

The girl's mother waved to me and said, "These special projects take a lot out of me! What a dreadful morning!"

If she only knew!

What do we see here? Poor motor coordination. Tactile overresponsivity. Sibling rivalry. Conflict between parents. Anger. Rage. Frustration. Loss of autonomy. Poor self-help skills. Passive aggression. Disorganization. Loss of self-control. Defiance. Helplessness. Despair. Guilt. Inadequacy. Isolation.

If you have an out-of-sync child, these problems may be all too familiar. The effects of SPD can permeate your lives.

Is it possible to learn to cope with the emotional fallout? Yes, if you understand your child, if you have support and understanding, and if you educate yourself.

Other Experts' Advice

Here are parenting techniques selected from the work of several child development experts, including Drs. A. Jean Ayres, Ross Greene, Stanley Greenspan, Mary Sheedy Kurcinka, Daniel Shapiro, Daniel Siegel, Larry Silver, Stanley Turecki, Sarah Wayland, and Serena Wieder. Their ideas may help you develop consistent and positive coping skills. (See www.out-of-sync -child.com for a current list of recommended books.)

PAY ATTENTION TO YOUR CHILD

Remember that the child's problem is a physical one. Just as another child with measles cannot help itching, the child with SPD cannot help being clumsy or afraid.

Tune in to the kinds of stimulation that the child avoids or craves.

Find the best way to reach your child, through his preferred sensory channel. Use a variety of ways to communicate (talking, writing, drawing, gesturing, and demonstrating). Keep your messages simple.

Identify your child's temperament by analyzing traits such as activity level, distractibility, intensity, regularity, sensory threshold, flexibility, and mood.

Know your child's strengths and weaknesses. If your child has been diagnosed, study the evaluations carefully. Get information from teachers and specialists who are familiar with differing abilities and learning styles. Take a look at "The Gander," a developmental-behavioral screening tool for parents, by Dan Shapiro, MD.[1]

Understand that most children with challenging behaviors usually have not one but a combination of several developmental differences, all at play simultaneously.

Sit on the floor and follow your child's play, paying attention to whatever interests him. Engaging with your child on his terms establishes a warm, trusting attachment, the basis of all future relationships. (Floortime was developed by Stanley Greenspan, MD, and Serena Wieder, PhD.)[2]

Identify the skills your child lacks for responding to your expectations. These skills may be flexibility and adaptability, frustration tolerance, and problem-solving.

Identify your child's challenging situations and behaviors at home, at school, in the community, and in relationships, to help you develop proactive strategies.

ANTICIPATE RESPONSES

Anticipate emotional crises. Too much stimulation at a birthday party or a crowded mall may trigger a negative response. Be ready to remove the child from sensations that will overwhelm her before she loses control.

Help the child learn to notice her increasing intensity and need for space. Give her opportunities to remove herself from the action and to recharge by being alone.

Develop strategies with your child to cope with negative emotions before they occur. "Let's lay out your clothes tonight, so in the morning you won't feel rushed."

To defuse her strong reactions, be prepared to provide soothing activities, such as a bath, story, quiet imaginative play, rocking chair, back rub, or outdoor play.

If she is slow to react to sensory stimuli, allow her extra time before responding.

EMPATHIZE

Identify and empathize with the child's point of view, motives, and goals to help you understand his behavior, so you will have an easier time changing it.

Understand the child's feelings and reflect them back: "It is hard to sleep when you are worried about the monster in the closet." Reflective listening helps him identify and master his emotions.

Reassure him repeatedly that you understand his difficulties.

Share your own similar emotions, to show that we all have fears. "I think roller coasters are scary, too" or "We both get nervous in crowds."

Continue talking to her about her experiences and her feelings about them. This will help her integrate the memories in her brain, develop emotional intelligence, and understand her own and others' feelings.

Take time to reevaluate your child's emotions. He may be aggressive because he is afraid, not angry. Respond to the primary emotion rather than to the defensive behavior.

Give your child coping skills for regaining self-control. After an emotional storm, provide a quiet space, a firm hug or a walk, or appropriate words or actions to restore harmony. "Do you need to do something to feel better about what happened?"

Accentuate the positive. Comment about his abilities, interests, and good behavior. Build his self-concept by reinforcing his growing self-awareness and accomplishments.

Build on his strengths and help him compensate for his weaknesses. Welcome him to the world; do not excuse him from life.

PROVIDE STRUCTURE

Establish consistent routines and schedules. Explain daily plans. Give notice of upcoming activities. Avoid surprises.

Limit transitions as much as possible. Allow time to end one activity before moving on to the next.

Expect the child to take longer than others to adapt to routines.

Help your child become organized in his own work. Together, set up schedules and job charts. Eliminate distractions. Provide sufficient space, time, and guidance to complete projects and homework so that he has the satisfaction of doing his work independently.

HAVE REALISTIC EXPECTATIONS

Sometimes, your child may function well, and other times, she will resist going to school, spill her milk, and fall. Expect inconsistency. When she stumbles, try to be understanding.

Break challenges into small pieces. Encourage her to achieve one goal at a time to feel the satisfaction of a series of little successes.

Remember that your child's brain will continue to develop into his mid-twenties. Until his brain has integrated more sensations and information about the world, his responses will naturally be less mature, logical, and reasonable than you may hope.

Remember that you have had years of experience in learning to deal with the world, and that the child has not.

DISCIPLINE

When the child loses control, avoid punishment. Loss of self-control is scary enough; punishment adds guilt and shame.

Comment on the child's negative behavior, not on the child: "Your yelling makes me angry" rather than "You infuriate me!"

Help the child find a quiet space, away from sensory overload, as a technique to regain self-control. Let him decide on the length of the time-out, if possible.

Set limits, to make a child feel secure. Pick one battle at a time to help him develop self-control and appropriate behavior.

Be firm about the limits you set. Show him that his feelings won't change the outcome; a rule is a rule. "I know you're mad because you want to play with the puppy, but it is suppertime."

Discipline consistently. Use gestures and empathy to explain why you are disciplining him. (Discipline means to teach or instruct, not punish.) After you tell him what you are going to do, then do it.

Determine appropriate consequences for misbehavior. A natural consequence is best, because it is reasonable and factual, and you do not impose it: "If you skip breakfast, you will be hungry." A logical consequence, in which the child is responsible for the outcome of his behavior, is second best: "If you throw the food, you must mop it up." An applied consequence, in which the punishment does not exactly fit the crime, is useful when nothing else works: "If you spit on the baby, you may not play with your friends" or "If you hit me, you may not watch TV."

Reward appropriate behavior with approval.

PROBLEM-SOLVE

Tackle the most important problems first. Begin with those that may be safety concerns.

Set up problem-solving time to discuss problems, negotiate differences, and arrive at solutions with your child. Elevating his problem-solving ability helps him anticipate challenges, take responsibility, cope with his feelings, become a logical and flexible thinker, and learn to compromise.

Ask him for advice on how you can help him. Collaborating to solve problems together makes you teammates, not opponents.

Help your child find appropriate outlets for emotions. Let her know when she can scream, where she can let loose, and what she can punch. Teach her that some negative expressions are acceptable and safe, while others are inappropriate.

When the child's intense emotions overwhelm you, first get control of your own feelings. You will show that strong emotions are a fact of life; everyone must learn to cope, and he, too, can learn to calm himself.

Have fun and laugh together. Life does not need to be serious all the time. Sharing a joke, funny video, or water-slide ride can dissolve tension and do a world of good.

If necessary, seek extra support to help with the "ripple effect" of your hard-to-raise child. Professionals can help you improve family life and relations with relatives, peers, and others outside of your nuclear family.

BECOME YOUR CHILD'S ADVOCATE

Educate adults who need to know about your child's abilities. Because SPD is invisible, people may forget or disbelieve that a significant problem affects your child. Your job is to inform them so that they can help your child learn.

Monitor your child's classroom and group activities. If you see that a teacher or coach is insensitive, uncooperative, or too demanding, take action.

Intervene when the child can't handle a stressful situation alone. Reinforce the message that asking for help is a positive coping strategy, not an admission of failure.

Dos and Don'ts for Coping

Here are my suggestions for dealing with the out-of-sync child on a daily basis.

WHAT TO DO

Do build on the child's strengths: "You are such a good cook! Help me remember what we need for our meat loaf recipe. Then you can mix it." Or, "You have energy to spare. Could you run over to Mrs. Johnson's house and get a magazine she has for me?" Think "ability," not "disability."

Do build on the child's interests: "Your collection of rocks is growing fast. Let's read some books about rocks. We can make a list of the different kinds you have found." Your interest and support will encourage the child to learn more and do more.

Do suggest small, manageable goals to strengthen your child's abilities: "How about if you walk with me just as far as the mailbox? You can drop the letter in. Then I'll carry you piggyback all the way home." Or, "You can take just one dish at a time to clear the table. We aren't in a hurry."

Do encourage self-help skills: To avoid "learned helplessness," sponsor your child's independence. "I know tying your shoes is hard, but each time you do it, it will get easier." Stress how capable she is, and how much faith you have in her, to build her self-esteem and autonomy. Show her you have expectations that she can help herself.

Do let your child engage in appropriate self-therapy: If your child craves spinning, let him spin on the tire swing with supervision. If he likes to jump on the bed, get him a trampoline or put a mattress on the floor. If he likes to hang upside down, install a chinning bar in his bedroom doorway. If he insists on wearing boots every day, let him wear boots. If he frequently puts inedible objects into his mouth, give him chewing gum. If he cannot sit still, give him opportunities to move and balance, such as sitting on a beach ball while he listens to music or a story. He will seek sensations that nourish his hungry brain, so help him find safe ways to do so.

Do offer new sensory experiences: "This lavender soap is lovely. Want to smell it?" Or, "Turnips crunch like apples but taste different. Want a bite?"

Do touch your child in ways that the child can tolerate and enjoy: "I'll rub your back with this sponge. Hard or gently?" Or, "Do you know what three quick hand squeezes mean, like this? I-love-you!"

Do encourage movement: "Let's swing our arms to the beat of this music. I always feel better when I stretch, don't you?" Movement always improves sensory processing.

Do encourage the child to try a new movement experience: "If you're interested in that swing, I'll help you get on."

Children with dyspraxia may enjoy new movement experiences but need help figuring out how to initiate them.

Do offer your physical and emotional support: "I'm interested in that swing. Want to try it with me? You can sit on my lap, and we'll swing together." The child who is fearful of movement may agree to swing at the playground if he has the security of a loving lap. (Stop if he resists.)

Do allow your child to experience unhappiness, frustration, or anger: "Wow, it really hurts when you don't get picked for the team." Acknowledging his feelings allows him to deal with them, whereas rushing in to make it better every time he's hurt prevents him from learning to cope with negative emotions.

Do provide appropriate outlets for negative emotions: Make it possible to vent pent-up feelings. Give her a ball or a bucketful of wet sponges to hurl against the fence. Designate a "screaming space" (her room, the basement, or the garage) where she can go to pound her chest and shout.

Do reinforce what is good about your child's feelings and actions, even when something goes wrong: "You didn't mean for the egg to miss the bowl. Cracking eggs takes practice. I'm glad you want to learn. Try again." Help her assess her experience positively by talking over what she did right and what she may do better the next time. How wonderful to hear that an adult is sympathetic rather than judgmental!

Do praise: "I noticed that you fed and walked the dog. Thanks for being so responsible." Reward the child for goodness, empathy, and being mindful of the needs of others. "You are a wonderful friend" or "You make animals feel safe."

Do give the child a sense of control: "If you choose bed now, we'll have time for a long story. If you choose to play longer, we won't have time for a story. You decide." Or, "I am ready to go to the shoe store whenever you are. Tell me when you're ready to leave." Impress on the child that others do not have to make every decision that affects him.

Do set reasonable limits: To become civilized, every child needs limits. "It is okay to be angry but not okay to hurt someone. We do not pinch."

Do recall how you behaved as a child: Maybe your child is just like you once were. (The apple doesn't fall far from the tree!) Ask yourself what you would have liked to make your childhood easier and more pleasurable. More trips to the playground, free time, or cuddling? Fewer demands? Lower expectations? Try saying, "When I was a kid and life got rough, I liked to climb trees. How about you?"

Do respect your child's needs even if they seem unusual: "You sure do like a tight tuck-in! There, now you're as snug as a bug in a rug." Or, "I'll stand in front of you while we're on the escalator. I won't let you fall."

Do respect your child's fears even if they seem senseless: "I see that your ball bounced near those big kids. I'll go with you. Let's hold hands." Your reassurances will help her trust others.

Do say "I love you": Assure your child that you accept and value who she is. You cannot say "I love you" too often!

Do follow your instincts: Your instincts will tell you that everyone needs to touch and be touchable, to move and be movable. If your child's responses seem atypical, ask questions, get information, and follow up with appropriate action.

Do listen when others express concerns: When teachers or caregivers suggest that your child's behavior is unusual, you may react with denial or anger. But remember that they see your child away from home, among many other children. Their perspective is worth considering.

Do educate yourself about typical child development: Read. Take parent-education classes. Learn about invariable stages of human development as well as variable temperaments and learning styles. It is comforting to know that a wide variety of behaviors falls within the normal range. Then you will find it easier to differentiate between typical and atypical behavior. Sometimes a cigar is just a cigar, and a six-year-old is just a six-year-old!

Do seek professional help: SPD is a problem that a child cannot overcome alone. Parents and teachers cannot "cure" a child, just as a child cannot cure himself.

Do keep your cool: When your child drives you crazy, collect your thoughts before responding, especially if you are angry, upset, or unpleasantly surprised. A child who is out of control needs the calm reassurance of someone who is in control. She needs a grown-up.

Do take care of yourself: When you're having a hard day, take a break! Hire a babysitter and go for a walk, read a book, take a bath, dine out, make love. Nobody can be expected to give another person undivided attention and still cope.

WHAT NOT TO DO

Don't try to persuade your child that he will outgrow his difficulties: "One day you will climb Mt. Everest!" Growing older does not always mean growing stronger, more agile, or more sociable. For children with SPD, growing older often means inventing new ways to avoid everyday experiences.

Don't tell your child she is bound to get stronger, better organized, or more in control if she applies herself: "You can do better if you'll just try!" The child is trying.

Don't joke: "Why are you so tired? Did you just run a

four-minute mile, ha ha?" Being tired is not a laughing matter to the child. Jokes make him feel laughed at and produce self-defeating anger and humiliation.

Don't plead: "Do it for Mommy. If you loved me, you'd sit up like a nice young lady." Your child does love you and yearns to please you, but she can't. Besides, she would sit up straight if she could, for her own sake, even if she didn't love you!

Don't shame: "A big boy like you can open the door all by himself." He may be big yet have little strength.

Don't threaten: "If you don't pick your feet up when you walk, then you'll ruin your shoes and you won't get any new ones." If/then threats backfire.

Don't talk about your child in demeaning ways in front of him: "This dopey-looking kid is my son. Wake up, lazy-bones, and give our new neighbor a high five!" Such comments are not funny to the listener.

Don't talk about your child in demeaning ways behind his back: "My kid is such a lazy good-for-nothing. I just can't get him to understand the importance of hard work." What do you want your boss, relatives, and friends to remember about your child?

Don't compare, aloud, one child with another: "Your brother rode a two-wheeler when he was six. What's wrong with you?" (But do note to yourself the abilities your child seems to lack, compared with others of the same age.)

Don't do for your child what your child can do for himself: "I'll sharpen your pencils while you get out your homework." Pampering a child gets you both nowhere fast.

Don't expect consistency: "You could hang your coat up yesterday. Why can't you do it today?" Inconsistency is common in out-of-sync children. What worked yesterday may not work today, and vice versa!

Don't make your child do things that distress him: "You must put your hand into this paint to make a handprint for Grandpa" or "You will love riding the elevator up in the Empire State Building." You cannot make him enjoy touch or movement experiences until his neurological system is ready.

Don't overload your child with multisensory experiences: "Let's eat some chili, put on some steel-band music, and dance the rumba. We're going to have a terrific south-of-the-border night." Slow down! Offering your child a variety of sensations, one at a time, is fine; offering her a variety of sensations, all at the same time, will overload her system.

Don't be afraid of "labeling" your child: Many parents fear the stigma attached to SPD. They don't want their son or daughter to be labeled as a child with special needs. That fear is normal, but it does not help your child. Consider the identification of SPD as a benefit, for now you know that your child can get help before the problem turns into a serious learning disability.

Don't feel helpless: The world is full of children with SPD and the people who love them. You and your child are not alone. Support is out there; it awaits you, and you can find it.

14

Looking at Your Child
in a New Light

A Parent's Epiphany

A father writes, "When I first heard the words 'sensory processing' and 'low muscle tone' used in connection with my daughter Julie, I both didn't know what they meant and also dismissed them as yet another example of my wife's overprotectiveness. These terms were used by Stanley Greenspan, MD—one of the city's (and country's) top child psychiatrists—whom we had consulted on Julie's sleep problems. Such technical jargon was testimony, in my mind, to the unspoken alliance that surely persisted between high-paid child experts and jittery mothers.

"True, at twelve months, Julie did flop around a little more than I would have expected (she did not yet crawl or stand), and true, she didn't snuggle as I had hoped. But I chalked it up to her being a little prickly and thought she was fine just as she was. The fact is, I hadn't seen enough other kids (as my wife and the doctor had) to know that her behavior was out of the ordinary.

"While I was either objecting or standing aside, my wife persisted. She took Julie to an occupational therapist—also well paid and ready to agree with the diagnosis—and put Julie into a twice-a-week course of therapy. I remained skeptical.

"The turning point came when I attended a workshop called Understanding Sensory Processing. While the presentation initially had limited impact on me, I was impressed with the number of parents who were there. 'So maybe this sensory stuff is for real,' I thought, 'and we're not the only ones who are concerned.'

"More important than the large turnout were the 'experience' stations in the back of the room. When I tried to accomplish simple tasks with some of my senses impaired—walking a straight line while looking through the wrong end of a pair of binoculars, for example—it started to penetrate my thick skull that Julie may in fact have entered the world with some special needs, and would have to compete with her peers at an unfair disadvantage as long as she had them.

"Suddenly, the significance of all this dawned on me—and I began to look at my daughter in a new light.

"From that point on, I became increasingly supportive of whatever would expand Julie's sensory and gross-motor horizons. I remember our glee when Julie started mashing food with her hands. I am now aghast that, out of ignorance and bravado, I would probably have denied Julie help at a critical time in her life, when she had her best chance to keep sensory deficiencies from becoming deep and lasting scars. And I applaud my wife, who was forced to do battle on two fronts—Julie's deficiencies and my resistance—to allow Julie to overcome her deficiencies before she ever knew she had them."

Becoming Enlightened

When you begin to understand SPD, you, too, will begin to look at your child in a new light. Recognizing that he is struggling to master the simplest tasks of everyday life is the first step toward helping him while he is still young.

Accepting your child's limitations is not easy. It is natural to want to deny that your child's difficulties are out of the ordinary. It is natural to feel sad when you understand how hard he must work. It is natural to feel guilty for the times you scolded him or got impatient because of his behavior.

It takes time to become enlightened. It will take psychic and physical energy to begin the journey toward making him feel better about himself and about what he can achieve. If you are reading this, you are already on the road, so take heart. It is going to get better.

Your child is unable, not unwilling, to perform routine tasks. Maybe she often says that she is "just too tired." Maybe she slumps over the dining room table instead of sitting upright, or hasn't the energy to turn a doorknob, although she seems to be eating and sleeping enough.

Redirect your thinking: When she says she's tired, she means it. She really is unable—not unwilling—to perform routine tasks. No matter how much she wants to be independent and peppy, her sensory processing differences hinder her motoric ability. She knows, subconsciously, that her strength is limited. She has deduced how to reserve it for the jobs she knows she must do, which may be chewing, getting in and out of the car, or bending down to retrieve a dropped spoon.

Your child is not lazy; in fact, she uses enormous energy just to get through the day.

Your child has developed some clever compensatory

skills. Away from home, it could be that your child does not appear to be as smart as you know he is. He may not talk much, giving the impression that he has little to discuss. Conversely, he may talk nonstop, yet be a poor conversationalist.

He may seem uncommonly shy with unfamiliar adults and other children. He may choose the same old games and toys, as if he lacks curiosity and a sense of intellectual adventure.

Redirect your thinking: SPD affects all kinds of children, including those who are extremely intelligent. Give your child credit for being so bright that he has figured out how to avoid making a fool of himself when he knows he cannot meet others' expectations.

Perhaps your child has lofty thoughts but cannot express them well because of a language disability that is sometimes associated with vestibular challenges. Or he may be verbally adept with a repertoire of excuses for evading intolerable movement or tactile experiences: "I can't paint today, because I'm wearing my new shirt and I shouldn't get it dirty."

Perhaps he has learned that if you see him digging in the sandbox, you will leave him alone. If he's busy, maybe you won't urge him to get on the swing, an activity that makes him feel that he is falling off the earth. You may notice that he looks up at you frequently, checking in for your approval, rather than concentrating on digging all the way to China.

Perhaps, if he cannot climb stairs easily, he has figured out a way to get you to carry him. When a child reaches up two small arms for an embrace and says, "Hug me up the stairs," what parent would believe that neurological differences are a problem?

Your child has developed compensatory skills that allow him to devise acceptable methods of avoiding the areas he knows will give him trouble.

Your child has courage. Perhaps your child resists descending the playground slide, does not like to play at other children's houses, shuns new foods, or becomes very anxious before visiting the doctor for an annual checkup. You may be exasperated by what you see as her excessive and inappropriate fearfulness.

Redirect your thinking: People need fear; fear alerts us to danger. Your child's apprehensions may seem excessive, but they are appropriate for her because her world seems dangerous. Each day she must face the same scary situations, such as a fear of losing her balance or of being touched. No wonder she is cautious about new situations, which are even scarier because they are unpredictable.

Furthermore, it takes courage to resist enjoyable experiences, resist change, or resist a parent. The penalty for disappointing an important grown-up is disapproval. No one seeks disapproval. But disapproval is preferable to proceeding with an activity that the child perceives as life-threatening.

Your child is brave, not a coward.

Your child has a tender heart. Perhaps your child has a "bad boy" reputation. He behaves aggressively, confronting the world with a stick in his hand, slugging the playmate who brushes against him, and shouting, "I hate that!" "This is boring!" "You're stupid!" "Get away or I'll kill you!" These antagonistic responses may make your child appear to be a truly unpleasant person, even if you know that within the bully beats a tender heart.

Redirect your thinking: Perhaps your child cannot differentiate between benign and hostile tactile experiences. Because he must protect himself from situations that he senses are dangerous, he instinctively chooses fight over flight. He puts up a

"Don't mess with me" façade not because he is misanthropic, but because he is scared.

The child who is inwardly on the defensive will often be outwardly offensive. An air of arrogance or a tough-guy image is common among people (adults, too) who feel uncertain about their abilities and self-worth.

You know how loving your child can be at home, in his familiar surroundings. He would be gentle outside the family circle, too, if he felt more comfortable in the world.

Your child has many abilities. Your child may not be skillful at reading, running, or paying attention. Her shortcomings may disappoint you.

Redirect your thinking: She may show extraordinary empathy and compassion for other living things. She may have a rare talent for creative thinking and be artistic, musical, or poetic. She may be observant where others are oblivious. She may have a wonderful sense of humor. Her special sensitivities may be a tremendous asset. Think abilities, not disabilities.

Your child has a special need for love and approval. Maybe she strikes you as being too possessive. She grabs all the toys but may not play with them; she just wants to have them. She demands all your time, but when you give it to her, she is unsatisfied. If she loses a round of Candy Land, she cries and mopes. She wants it all.

Redirect your thinking: She requires things and attention to bolster her own small store of self-esteem. She has to be the winner because she usually feels like a loser. She seems greedy because she is needy.

More than anything, your child has a special need to be loved and appreciated.

Your child's "hardheadedness" is a survival skill.

Perhaps he says things like "I'm the boss of my own body. You can't tell me what to do." Perhaps he is rigid, always wanting to wear the same clothes and eat the same cereal in the same bowl. Perhaps he insists on elaborate rituals for bath- or bedtime.

Redirect your thinking: Nobody awakens in the morning thinking, "Today I'm going to resist everything." Human beings learn to cope with a changing environment by being flexible. Your little fellow appears stubborn, however, because he is not the boss of his own body, and he is not in control. His life is full of uncertainties and obstacles.

An inefficient tactile system, with an attendant fussiness about clothing, may be the reason that he wants to wear shorts when it snows. Because the inside of his mouth may be overly sensitive to food textures, he may insist on the same kind of cereal, day after day.

Sameness and rituals are tools that help him accomplish basic jobs, like getting dressed or preparing for bed. His apparent stubbornness is rooted in his need to survive.

He is not willfully stubborn; he is stubborn because he has trouble adapting his behavior to meet changing demands, so he sticks to what he knows will work.

Your child truly requires your attention, tailored to his needs. Let's suppose you dress your little boy in the morning, because he takes so long and becomes tearfully frustrated when you leave the job up to him. Then let's suppose that his teacher mentions how much extra time is required for her to attend to his needs. She suggests that you urge him to become independent in the getting-dressed department. Even if you know more than she does about problems caused by SPD, you may still believe that your parenting skills are inadequate.

Redirect your thinking: Giving your child attention when

he needs it and when a job must get done quickly is perfectly okay. Particularly when your family runs on a tight schedule, you will do whatever works to move everybody from point A to point B.

Unenlightened parents ignore their children. Enlightened parents do what they can to make their children's lives pleasant and safe.

Your child can function better—with help. If your child has sensory processing difficulties now, her problems will grow with her. Certainly, she may develop strategies to avoid or compensate for stressful sensory experiences. Certainly, she may develop talents that are not dependent upon her shaky sense of balance or hypersensitivity to touch. But she will always have to work very, very hard to function smoothly.

Redirect your thinking: SPD is like indigestion of the brain. Just as antacid can soothe upset stomachs, so can occupational therapy and a sensory-enriched life smooth neural pathways.

Most of all, your everyday love and empathy will boost your child's emotional security. We all need to know that someone is there for us, especially when times are rough.

A Parent's Encouraging Words

A mother writes: "If we had only known. If only there had been a book like this to read. If only our long- and eagerly awaited child had been 'normal.'

"Initially, we thought he was. He had great Apgar scores [measuring a newborn's condition] and was on schedule with all the developmental checklists. Certainly, he had no obvious physical abnormalities; he was beautiful. Moreover, he was alert, learning to talk at six months! When he was two years old, all the pediatricians at the clinic dropped what they were doing to observe his phenomenal verbal skills. We were so proud.

"But at the same time, we knew that something was not right. Something had not been right all along. In the newborn nursery, he cried so loudly that he kept all the other babies awake. Then there was the traumatic transition from breast to bottle feeding. In fact, any kind of transition from one experience to another was horrendous.

"He was also extremely sensitive to light touch and new textures. It was difficult to dress him. Then came a toddlers' gymnastics program, with terror and screaming at physical activities the other children loved. I had to face the stares from critical instructors and parents of more 'cooperative' children. With time, his behavior became more and more troublesome.

"What was wrong with my child? My beautiful and funny child.

"Finally, I contacted the public school's early childhood screening program, and we were scheduled for a group screening.

"When we arrived at the appointed time and place, we found many children with obvious handicaps and a play table to occupy them until it was their turn to go through the stations. Those with cognitive disabilities, braces, and missing limbs went ahead smoothly.

"At our turn, the transition from play to screening activity resulted in a screaming, limp child who could not be handled by all the experts assembled. We left in tears. Our son, the only child with no discernible problem, could not even be tested.

"Upon subsequent individual evaluation by a team including an educational specialist, occupational therapist, speech pathologist, and psychologist, we were finally introduced to the 'something wrong.' Its name was sensory processing disorder. It required 'occupational therapy' and 'a good nursery school.'

"Why had it taken so long? Why hadn't anyone known? Why had my family suffered so much?

"It didn't matter now. The good nursery school was at hand.

"Upon the recommendation of the evaluation team, I contacted St. Columba's. I will never forget my first conversation with Carol Kranowitz. It was the first day my fear began to abate. She was the music and movement teacher, but she was so much more. She was the first person to whom I had ever spoken who knew my child without ever having met him. That is because she knew about SPD and had undertaken to inform and train other staff in its idiosyncrasies and, even more important, its management.

"These people at St. Columba's were not afraid of my child. They didn't see him as 'bad' or 'uncontrolled.' They saw him struggling with sensory processing problems, and though he challenged them mightily, they never gave up.

"With occupational therapy, we began to overcome such hurdles as fear of movement and revulsion caused by unfamiliar textures. As his fear of new things diminished, as the world became a less scary place, transitions also improved. With a psychologist's help, we structured the environment and managed behavioral responses (i.e., tantrums) consistently.

"Gradually, our child has blossomed and we have learned to do something with him that I never thought would be possible. We learned to enjoy him. He is our favorite companion.

"As I look back upon two years of OT and a nurturing nursery school, I shudder to think what a mess we would all have been without them. They were our lifeline, our hold on hope.

"Here is my charge to you: If you have concerns about your own or another child, no matter how vague they seem or how inarticulate you feel verbalizing them, pursue them. A child can have less pronounced problems than mine and still need help. And in your pursuit, continue until you find hope. In doing so, you may free other wonderful, enjoyable little people held hostage by SPD. They are too small and frightened to free themselves."

Dear Reader: We all need to know that someone applauds our strengths, understands our challenges, and honors our individuality. With your knowledge about sensory processing and sensory processing differences, and with your loving support, your child can flourish and grow to become in sync with the world.

Appendix A

The Sensory Processing Machine

Here is a brief anatomy lesson about the central nervous system and an explanation of how sensory processing occurs therein. This overview may help you appreciate the marvel of the brain-and-body connection.

The Synchronized Nervous System

All animals respond to sensations of touch, movement and gravity, and body position. Thus, human animals share the hidden senses with goldfish and goats, falcons and frogs, caterpillars and clams. Through eons of evolution, humankind refined these senses in order to survive in a hazardous world.

As life-forms gradually arose from sea to land to treetops, they had to adapt to differing environments. Hands to pluck berries, limbs to climb trees, eyes to see moving as well as stationary objects, and ears to detect prey and predators developed over time.

Along with these skills came increasingly complex sensations. The human brain evolved to process these sensations so that the hand would pick a berry rather than a thorn, the limb would cling to a branch, the eye would discern a motionless tiger poised to pounce, and the ear would hear faraway hoofbeats.

With the most complex brain in the animal kingdom, humans have the most complex nervous system. Its main task is to process sensations.

The nervous system has three main parts, working in harmony. One is the peripheral nervous system, running through organs and muscles, such as the eyes, ears, and limbs. The second part is the autonomic nervous system, controlling the involuntary functions of heart rate, breathing, digestion, and reproduction. The third part is the central nervous system (CNS), consisting of numerous neurons, a spinal cord, and a brain.

Three Components of the Central Nervous System

A. THE NEURONS

Neurons, or nerve cells, are the structural and functional units of the nervous system. Neurons tell us what is happening inside and outside our bodies. The brain has approximately 86 billion neurons. Each neuron has:

- A cell body, with its nucleus inside.
- Many short dendrites (Greek for "little branches") reaching out to other neurons to receive messages, or impulses, and carrying them into the cell body.
- A long axon, like a stem with roots, which sends impulses from the cell body to the dendrites of other neurons.

Two kinds of neurons connect the brain and spinal cord to the rest of the body: sensory and motor. Sensory neurons receive impulses from sensory receptors in our eyes, ears, skin, muscles, joints, and organs.

Impulses travel along the sensory neuron's axon and communicate messages to other neurons at contact points called synapses (Greek for "point of juncture"). Each neuron makes thousands of synaptic connections every time it fires. The neuron firing off the message is called presynaptic; the neuron receiving the message is called postsynaptic.

At the nanosecond that the message is fired, neurotransmitters are released, causing an electrochemical response. When neurotransmitters activate the receptors of the postsynaptic neurons, they are called excitatory. When they do not activate receptors, they are called inhibitory. (The process of balancing excitatory and inhibitory messages is called modulation. See page 72.)

A NEURON

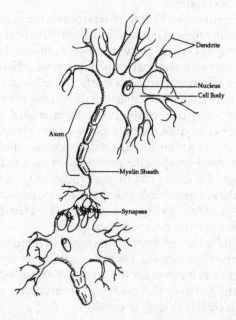

The postsynaptic neurons may be other sensory neurons, or they may be motor neurons, the second kind of neurons in our CNS. Receiving the information, the motor neurons instruct muscles to move, glands to sweat, lungs to breathe, intestines to digest, and other body parts to respond appropriately.

In the growing fetus, neurons and synaptic connections multiply rapidly. A baby is born with billions of neurons and trillions of synapses. Sensations of smell, touch, and hunger activate synaptic connections to help the baby survive. For instance, synaptic connections help him respond to a nipple so that he can suck.

To help the baby respond efficiently to this early skill of sucking, as well as to more complex skills, a process called myelination occurs. Myelin is a substance—somewhat like an electrical insulator—that coats the axon of the neuron to protect it, to smooth the path, and to speed up the connections.

At about eighteen months, the development of new neurons decreases to a trickle, because the child's brain now has almost all that it needs. New synapses, however, keep multiplying as the child integrates new sensations.

That is, synapses multiply if synaptic connections are useful for everyday functioning and repeatedly used. Otherwise, they vanish. If a person does not engage in a wide range of sensory experiences, using certain synaptic connections becomes more difficult. For instance, when astronauts return to Earth after a few days in outer space, they have trouble reestablishing their sense of balance, because their gravity receptors were not being stimulated.

By about twelve years, the child will lose many synapses he was born with, through a normal and necessary process called pruning. Pruning eliminates synapses the child does not need and stabilizes those he does. If a child's culture uses chopsticks, his brain will strengthen the synapses needed for that complex, one-handed motor skill. If his culture uses spoons and forks, his brain will prune the unnecessary connections for chopstick use.

Normally, as the child actively responds to sensations, useful synaptic connections increase. The more connections, the more myelination; the more myelination, the stronger the neurological structure; and the stronger the neurological structure, the better equipped the child is to learn new skills.

Two Examples of the Function of Neurotransmitters

City Sensations Become Routine

You leave your quiet country home and visit the city for the first time. The sound of traffic, the sight of crowds, the smell of pollution, and the motion of escalators bombard your senses. Billions of neurons are firing messages; zillions of neurotransmitters are activating neuronal responses. Your nervous system is operating on overtime; that is why you are so "nervous"!

After a few days, you begin to grow accustomed to city sensations. You no longer jump each time you hear screeching brakes or get jostled on the subway. Neurotransmitters now have less of an excitatory effect and more of an inhibitory effect. As your nervous system adapts to repeated stimuli, you can pay less attention to every sensation—and still survive.

Painkillers Become Less Effective

You have chronic back pain, so you take a painkiller. At first, the medicine helps as the neurotransmitters activate a response. After a while, the medicinal effect wears off because postsynaptic neurons have raised their threshold. Instead of just one painkiller to make you comfortable, you now require two or three.

B. THE SPINAL CORD

Extending below the brain is the spinal cord, a long, thick structure of nervous tissue. It receives all sensations from peripheral nerves in our skin and muscles and relays these messages up to the brain. The brain then interprets the sensory messages and sends motor messages back down to the spinal cord, which sends messages out to peripheral nerves in specific body parts.

C. THE BRAIN

The human brain evolved over the course of 500 million years. Dr. Paul D. MacLean, who was a brain researcher at the National Institute of Mental Health, proposed that each human is born with a "triune brain." (This model of brain development is one of many. For our purposes, it is the simplest.)

As we evolved, we added layers of brain material, each one improving earlier parts. The first layer is the reptilian complex: the "primitive brain." It is responsible for reflexive, instinctive functions necessary for self-preservation and sexual drive. Sometimes these functions are called the "Four F's": feeding, fighting, fleeing . . . and sexual reproduction.

The second layer is the limbic (Latin for "border") system. It is the "seat of emotions," controlling hormones that enable us to feel angry, lustful, and jealous, as well as pleased and happy. Sometimes

THE TRIUNE BRAIN

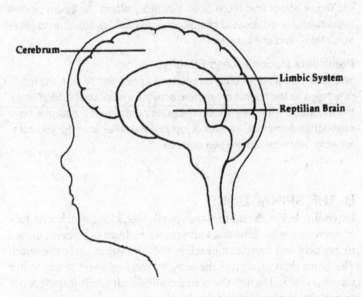

called the "smell brain," this system processes smell and taste, which have a powerful effect on our emotions.

The limbic system adds feelings to the otherwise instinctive behavior. Thus, when we feel threatened, we fight or flee—or shut down. When we feel safe, we can play—and when we play, we can learn.

The third layer is the cerebrum: the "thinking brain." It is responsible for the organization of the most complex sensory intake. Detailed processing of sensations occurs here, so we can think, remember, make decisions, solve problems, plan and execute our actions, and communicate through language.

Four Brain Parts Used in Sensory Processing

Four important brain structures are involved in sensory processing. Let's glance at them and see how they fit into the triune brain.

1. THE BRAIN STEM

The brain stem, part of the primitive brain, is an extension of the spinal cord. The brain stem performs four key functions.

- **A crossroads,** it receives sensory messages, particularly from skin and muscles in the head and neck, and relays this information to the cerebrum. In turn, the cerebrum sends out messages for motor coordination.

- **A switching gate,** it is the location where sensations from the left side of the body cross over to the right cerebral hemisphere, and vice versa. It is here that outgoing responses from the left hemisphere instruct the right side of the body what to do, and vice versa.

- **A clearinghouse,** it processes vestibular sensations necessary for hearing, maintaining our balance, seeing moving objects, and focusing our attention on one thing or another.

- **A regulator,** it processes sensations from internal organs and controls breathing, heartbeat, and digestion. It is the seat of the reticular core, a neuronal network that exchanges data with the vestibular system to guide our sense of timing for waking up, falling asleep, getting excited, and calming down.

A CROSS-SECTION OF THE BRAIN

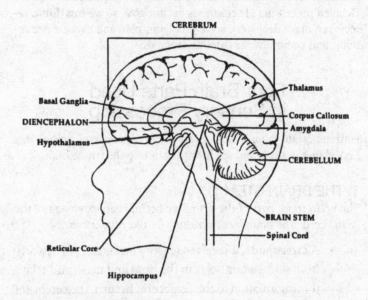

2. THE CEREBELLUM

Another part of the primitive brain is the cerebellum (Latin for "little brain"). Processing proprioceptive and vestibular sensations, it coordinates muscle tone, balance, and all our body movements. It controls fine-motor skills, especially repetitive movements, such as touch-typing and practicing scales. It lets us move easily, precisely, and with good timing. An Olympic diver has a finely tuned cerebellum that allows him to execute a seemingly effortless dive.

3. THE DIENCEPHALON

The diencephalon (Greek for "divided brain"), sometimes called the "tweenbrain," nestles in the center of the brain. A part of the limbic system, the diencephalon is associated with several important structures.

The basal ganglia (from Greek for "base of knots") are clusters of nerves that coordinate vestibular sensations necessary for balance and voluntary movement. The basal ganglia relay messages among the inner ear, the cerebellum, and the cerebrum.

The hippocampus (Greek for "sea horse," which it resembles) compares old and new stimuli. If it remembers a sensation, like the feel of comfortable shoes, it sends out inhibitory neurons to tell the cortex not to get aroused. If the sensation is new, like too-tight boots, it alerts the cortex with excitatory neurons.

The amygdala (Greek for "almond") connects impulses from the olfactory system and the cortex. It processes emotional memories, such as the smell of an old boyfriend's cologne, and influences emotional behavior, especially anger.

The hypothalamus (Greek for "under the inner chamber") controls the autonomic nervous system, regulating temperature, water metabolism, reproduction, hunger and thirst, and our state of alertness. It also has centers for emotions: anger, fear, pain, and pleasure.

The thalamus (Greek for "inner chamber") is the key relay station for processing all sensory data except smell. Most sensations pass through it en route to our great gift, the cerebrum.

4. THE CEREBRUM

The most recently developed layer of the triune brain is the cerebrum (Latin for "brain"). Its wrinkled surface is the cerebral cortex (Latin for "bark"), often referred to as the neocortex because it is new, in evolutionary terms. The cerebrum is composed of two cerebral hemispheres.

Why do we need two hemispheres? One theory is that the right and left hemispheres developed when early humanoids lived in trees and learned to use one hand independently from the other. This was a useful survival skill: one hand could gather fruit while the other clung to a branch. Asymmetric use of the hands and asymmetric hemispheres in the brain developed together in a process called lateralization (from Latin for "side").

With lateralization came specialization. Specialization describes the different jobs of the two hemispheres. With discrete duties, the right and left hemispheres must work together for us to function at a high level.

In general, the left hemisphere is the cognitive side. It directs analytical, logical, and verbal tasks, such as doing math and using language. It controls the right side of the body, which is usually the action-oriented side.

In general, the right hemisphere is the sensory, intuitive side. It directs nonverbal activities, such as recognizing faces, visualizing the shape of a pyramid, and responding to music. It controls the left side of the body.

The corpus callosum (Latin for "hard-skinned body"), a bundle of billions of nerve fibers, connects the hemispheres. This neural highway carries messages back and forth, and integrates the memories, perceptions, and responses that each hemisphere processes separately. Thus, our right hemisphere creates an original thought or tune, and our left lets us write it down. Our right and left eyes look at someone and see a whole person, not two separate halves. Our right hand knows what our left hand is doing.

Four Major Cortical Lobes

Each hemisphere has its own set of four major cortical lobes. Each lobe has a right side and a left side, both of which must work together, relaying neural messages back and forth, in order for the complex task of specialization to occur. The lobes have many administrative duties.

The occipital (Latin for "back of the skull") lobes are for vision. They begin to process visual images before sending them to the parietal and temporal lobes for further interpretation.

The parietal (Latin for "wall") lobes are for body sense. They process proprioceptive messages, so we sense the position of our body in space, and tactile messages such as pain, temperature, and touch discrimination. These lobes interact with other brain parts to give the "whole picture." For instance, they receive visual messages from the occipital lobes and integrate them with auditory and tactile messages, thus aiding vision and spatial awareness.

The temporal (Latin for "time") lobes are for hearing, for interpreting music and language, for refining vestibular sensations, and for memory.

The frontal lobes are for executive thinking. They have a motor area for organizing voluntary body movement and a prefrontal area concerned with aspects of personality—speech, reasoning, remembering, self-control, problem-solving, and planning ahead.

THE LEFT HEMISPHERE, SHOWING THE CORTICAL LOBES, SENSORY CORTEX, AND MOTOR CORTEX

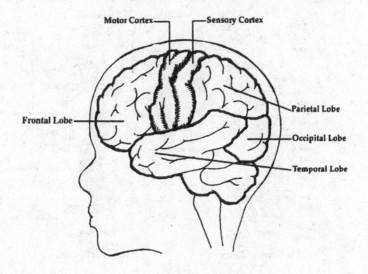

The Sensory Cortex and the Motor Cortex

Lying on the top are strips called the sensory cortex and the motor cortex. The sensory cortex receives tactile and proprioceptive sensations from the body. The motor cortex sends messages through peripheral nerves to the muscles.

In the early twentieth century, a Canadian neurosurgeon, Wilder Penfield, studied these cortical areas to learn about neural functions. The "maps" below (see page 338), based on his research, seem comically out of proportion. Their purpose is serious, however: to illustrate the relative importance of our body parts.

Considerable portions of the sensory cortex are dedicated to receiving messages from the head and the hands—more than from the torso or the arm, for instance. The reason is that body function is more important than body size; the head and hands have the most complex functions and thus produce the most sensations. Similarly large portions of the motor cortex are devoted to

PENFIELD'S MAPS

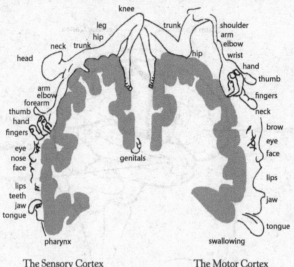

The Sensory Cortex   The Motor Cortex

*Illustrating how the sensory cortex and motor cortex assign specific areas
to different body parts, according to their relative importance.*

sending messages to direct the functions of the fingers, hands,
tongue, and throat.

Cerebral Hemispheres Make Us Human

Our cerebral hemispheres permit us to learn human skills, such as
the ability to stand upright, thereby freeing our hands for manipulating and carrying objects. They enable us to speak, to reason, and
to use symbols, thus enabling humankind to develop culture. They
allow us to remember the past and to plan for the future, thereby
increasing our chances for survival. They give us the mental tools
not only to react but also to "pro-act," that is, to anticipate what will
happen next and to prepare an appropriate response. The locus of
our finest movements and loftiest thoughts, they make us human.

Three Examples of How the Central Nervous System Processes Sensations

The Paper Cut

Working at the copy machine, you get a paper cut on your finger. Tactile receptors in your skin send the message via myelinated sensory neurons through your peripheral nervous system to your brain: up your arm, through your spinal cord to your brain stem, to your thalamus, to the sensory cortex. The sensory cortex analyzes the message and tells neurotransmitters to fire excitatory impulses.

First you become aware of the sense of light-touch pressure; a millisecond later, you are conscious of the tissue-damaging pain. Meanwhile, motor neurons send impulses to your finger. You say "Ouch!" and pull your finger away from the paper.

The Fall from the Ladder

Perched on a ladder, you stretch to paint the ceiling. Your triune brain is totally involved: cerebrum, as you plan the next stroke; limbic system, as you smell the paint and remember your first painting experience with Dad; and reptilian complex, as you improve your "nest."

You tilt your chin up a little higher, and your inner ear sends messages to your brain stem about this change of neck and head position. The brain stem relays the vestibular information to your cerebellum, basal ganglia, thalamus, and cerebrum.

Suddenly you feel dizzy, because your head is far off-center. You lose your balance, drop the paint can, and tumble to the floor.

Your hypothalamus registers that you are hurt, afraid, and angry. It alerts your autonomic nervous system to increase your heart rate and to sweat.

You lie in a heap. You cannot think about the spilling paint; when you feel endangered, your cerebrum shuts down and the reptilian brain takes over. Your instinct is self-preservation, so you wait until your reticular core calms you down. Regaining control, you realize that you are bruised but not broken. You arise and get busy.

The Car-Door Maneuver

Your arms are full of packages and you must close the car door. Your parietal and occipital lobes exchange information to help you gauge your spatial relationship to the car and to plan and execute the maneuver.

Motor neurons send messages through your cerebellum and spinal cord to muscles in your right leg. Excitatory neurons activate muscles on the back of your thigh, instructing them to flex. Inhibitory neurons activate muscles on the front of your thigh, instructing them to extend. Motor planning enables you to bend your knee and lift your right leg.

Meanwhile, the opposite happens in your left leg, which straightens. You stabilize your body and keep your balance.

Proprioceptors in your legs tell your brain what's happening. You push your right foot against the car door and slam it shut.

The Sensory Processing Machine: Summary

This discussion of the sensory processing machine demonstrates the crucial interrelationship of the central nervous system and the senses. It also shows that all parts of the central nervous system must communicate in order to process senses.

It is critical to understand that no matter how much advanced brain power a child has, intelligence alone is not sufficient for organized, daily functioning if the underlying senses are not in good working order. A child's smooth development depends on smooth sensory processing.

Appendix B

Dr. Ayres's Four Levels of Sensory Integration

In *Sensory Integration and the Child,* Dr. Ayres described the development of functional skills as the "Four Levels of Integration." As you read this summary, please refer to the building blocks illustration on page 83.

Level One (Primary Sensory Systems)

The infant busily takes in sensory information, establishing the foundation for all future learning. While the visual, auditory, and other senses are operating, the primary "teachers" are skin (the tactile sense), gravity and movement (the vestibular sense), and muscles (the proprioceptive sense).

Touch stimulation feels good on his skin and around his mouth (an extremely sensitive tactile receptor). He sucks with pleasure and enjoys being held and rocked. A strong feeling of attachment develops as a result of this sensory connection between mother and child. The baby learns that eating, cuddling, and being friendly provide positive feedback.

Through his vestibular and proprioceptive senses, the baby receives information about his movement. He begins to regulate his eye movements, too. He blinks when a speck of dust approaches his eye. With his budding visual sense, he can see motionless objects nearby as well as people and things moving around him. He anticipates and imitates his mother's facial expressions. He learns to rely on the comings and goings of the people near him.

Vestibular and proprioceptive senses also affect his posture and muscle tone. He tries new movements and, after some effort, succeeds. He lifts his head against gravity, then his shoulders, and, arching up with his weight on his hands and abdomen, he pivots on his stomach and looks around. He hears Mommy sing his name and turns to greet her. Moving in response to the environment is effective. The more he moves, the more confident he becomes.

Vestibular sensations about gravity, coming through his inner ear, teach him that he is connected to the earth. He feels safe.

Level Two (Sensory-Motor Skills)

Having processed basic senses at Level One, the toddler begins to develop body awareness. This is a mental picture of where body parts are, how they interrelate, and how they move. Visual feedback adds to a sense of self.

Along with body awareness comes bilateral (two-sided) integration. This is the process that enables the child to use both sides of her body symmetrically, in a smooth, simultaneous, and coordinated way.

Bilateral integration, a neurological process, is the foundation for bilateral coordination, an emerging perceptual-motor skill. Bilateral coordination is necessary for such interesting work as passing a rattle back and forth from hand to hand.

A function of bilateral integration is lateralization, the process of establishing preference of one side of the brain for directing efficient movement on the opposite side of the body.

Postural responses improve. The child can get into and stay in different positions. She develops neck stability and can raise her head and torso to look around.

Neck stability helps the eyes hold steady so the child can gaze at whatever interests her. In turn, stabilization of the eyes helps the child improve motor control, for the more she uses her eyes to observe her surroundings, the more she coordinates her movements.

With developing binocularity, or eye teaming, she looks where she is going and goes where she is looking.

She begins to crawl on her stomach, then creep on all fours. As she alternates her hands and legs, she uses both sides of her brain and stimulates bilateral coordination.

Her maturing tactile, vestibular, and proprioceptive senses promote praxis, or motor planning. She can figure out how to do something she has never done before and then do it again. Rolling over, for example, requires motor planning the first few times, until the child has practiced it so often that she can roll over effortlessly.

Practicing sensory-motor skills all day long means that the child's activity level becomes better regulated. Her attention span and emotional security increase because her sensations are becoming well organized. She can sit in her car seat for a ride to the grocery store. She can bang on the piano keys for a few minutes. She can fall asleep peacefully at the end of her busy day.

Level Three (Perceptual-Motor Skills)

As the child develops, so does cognitive understanding of the information that his senses take in. As sensory discrimination improves, his ability to interact with the external world broadens.

Hearing (the auditory sense) becomes more refined. He can understand language and communicate through speech.

Vision becomes more precise. He can interpret visual data more accurately. He understands spatial relationships and can discriminate where people and objects are and where he is in relation to them.

Bilateral coordination improves with continuous movements using both sides of the body. The child develops laterality and begins to demonstrate a hand preference, uses his hands separately, and crosses the midline.

Eye-hand coordination develops. Now the child can hold a crayon, draw a simple picture, catch a ball, and pour juice. Eye-hand coordination contributes to visual-motor integration, necessary for such tasks as putting together a string of pop beads or fitting a jigsaw puzzle piece into place.

Indeed, the child can do a jigsaw puzzle now—just for the fun of it—with purposeful, playful activity. When he picks up a jigsaw piece, it is his developing sensory processing that lets him see it, handle it, understand it, and fit it into the puzzle.

As a preschooler, the child continues to develop and strengthen basic skills. Now he is ready for the top block—the end products of sensory processing, on Level Four.

Level Four (Academic Readiness)

The end products of sensory integration are academic skills (including abstract thought and reasoning), complex motor skills, regulation of attention, organization of behavior, specialization of each side of the body and the brain, visualization, self-esteem, and self-control.

These abilities become increasingly sophisticated. By kindergarten or first grade, the child's brain is mature enough to specialize. Specialization (the process whereby one brain part becomes most efficient at a particular function) means that the child becomes more efficient and purposeful in her actions. Her eyes and ears are prepared to take over as the primary "teachers."

She can suppress reflexive responses to unexpected touch sensations and her tactile discrimination improves. Outdoors on a wintry day, she can ignore the minor discomfort of an itchy wool hat and concentrate on making a snowball. She can tell the difference between a friendly pat and an aggressive punch.

Her proprioceptive sense, in tandem with her vestibular and tactile senses, strengthens her motor coordination. Her gross-motor skills are smooth: She can jump and run and play with her pals.

Her fine-motor skills are good: She can button, zip, and spin a top. She consistently prefers to use one hand more than the other for tool use. She controls a pencil or crayon to make recognizable shapes and symbols.

She can visualize past and future situations: yesterday's ball game and tonight's bath. Visualization helps her picture pretend and real images: make-believe monsters and Mommy's reassuring face.

She is socially competent, able to share ideas and toys, to be flexible when things do not go her way, to empathize with others when things do not go their way, to play by the rules, to be a reliable friend.

The child will continue to process sensations throughout her life. As she encounters different situations and new challenges, she learns to make adaptations in meaningful ways. With a well-established sense of self, she is ready for school and the big world.

Notes

Introduction

1. L. A. Balzer-Martin and C. S. Kranowitz (1987). *The Balzer-Martin Preschool Screening.* Available from St. Columba's Nursery School, in Washington, DC, (202) 742-1980, or https://stcolumbasnursery school.org.

A Word About Words and That Pesky "D" in "SPD"

1. A. J. Ayres (2005). *Sensory Integration and the Child: Understanding Hidden Sensory Challenges.* Los Angeles: Western Psychological Services, 3.
2. S. Smith Roley, Z. Mailloux, H. Miller-Kuhaneck, and T. Glennon (2007). "Understanding Ayres' Sensory Integration." *OT Practice*, 12(7).
3. L. J. Miller, M. Anzalone, S. Lane, S. A. Cermak, and E. Osten (2007). "Concept Evolution in Sensory Integration: A Proposed Nosology for Diagnosis." *American Journal of Occupational Therapy*, 61, 135–40.
4. L. J. Miller, S. Schoen, S. Mulligan (unpublished manuscript). *Sensory Processing Three Dimensions Scale Manual (SP3D).* Torrance, CA: Western Psychological Services.

Chapter Two: Does Your Child Have Sensory Processing Differences?

1. Miller et al. (2007). "Concept Evolution in Sensory Integration."
2. D. Shapiro (2016). *Parent Child Journey*, 10–15. "The Gander" screening tool, designed by Dr. Dan Shapiro with contributions from Sarah Wayland, is also available at www.parentchildjourney .com/wp-content/uploads/2016/11/Your-Gander-Instruction -Manual-11.26.2016.pdf.

3. K. Mahler (2015). *Interoception: The Eighth Sensory System.* Lenexa, KS: AAPC Publishing, 31.

4. C. S. Kranowitz (2016). *The Out-of-Sync Child Grows Up: Coping with Sensory Processing Disorder in the Adolescent and Young Adult Years.* New York: TarcherPerigee, 93.

5. A. M. Davis, A. S. Bruce, R. Khasawneh, T. Schulz, C. Fox, and W. Dunn (2013). "Sensory Processing Issues in Young Children Presenting to an Outpatient Feeding Clinic: A Retrospective Chart Review." *Journal of Pediatric Gastroenterology and Nutrition,* 56(2), 156–60.

6. Kranowitz (2016). *The Out-of-Sync Child Grows Up,* 140.

7. R. V. Whitney and W. Pickren (2014). *Self-Regulation: A Family Systems Approach for Children with Autism, Learning Disabilities, ADHD, and Sensory Disorders.* Eau Claire, WI: PESI Publishing & Media, passim.

8. R. Ahn, L. J. Miller, S. Milberger, and D. N. McIntosh (2004). "Prevalence of Parents' Perceptions of Sensory Processing Disorders among Kindergarten Children." *American Journal of Occupational Therapy,* 58(3), 287–302.

9. A. Ben-Sasson, A. S. Carter, and M. J. Briggs-Gowan (2009). "Sensory Over-Responsivity in Elementary School: Prevalence and Social-Emotional Correlates." *Journal of Abnormal Child Psychology,* 37(5), 705–16.

Chapter Three: Does Your Child Have Another Diagnosis?

1. Ben-Sasson et al. (2009). "Sensory Over-Responsivity in Elementary School."

2. M. L. Danielson, R. H. Bitsko, R. M. Ghandour, J. R. Holbrook, M. D. Kogan, and S. J. Blumberg (2018). "Prevalence of Parent-Reported ADHD Diagnosis and Associated Treatment among U.S. Children and Adolescents, 2016." *Journal of Clinical Child & Adolescent Psychology,* 47(2), 199–212.

3. Ahn, et al. (2004). "Prevalence of Parents' Perceptions."

4. M. J. Maenner, K. A. Shaw, J. Baio, A. Washington, M. Patrick, M. DiRienzo, D. L. Christensen, et al. (2020). "Prevalence of Autism Spectrum Disorder among Children Aged 8 Years—Autism and Developmental Disabilities Monitoring Network, 11 Sites, United States, 2016." *Centers for Disease Control and Prevention: Morbidity and Mortality Weekly Report—Surveillance Summaries,* 69(4), 1–12.

5. S. D. Tomcheck and W. Dunn (2007). "Sensory Processing in Children with and without Autism: A Comparative Study Using the

Short Sensory Profile." *American Journal of Occupational Therapy*, 61(2), 190–200.

6. T. F. Boat and J. T. Wu, eds. (2015). "Prevalence of Learning Disabilities." Chapter 16 in *Mental Disorders and Disabilities among Low-Income Children*. Washington, DC: National Academies Press, 281–94.

7. Individuals with Disabilities Education Act, or IDEA 04 (2004). 20 U.S.C. § 1400.

8. E. J. Marco (2021). Personal communication.

9. Ahn et al. (2004). "Prevalence of Parents' Perceptions."

10. L. J. Miller, D. M. Nielsen, and S. A. Schoen (2012). "Attention Deficit Hyperactivity Disorder and Sensory Modulation Disorder: A Comparison of Behavior and Physiology." *Research in Developmental Disabilities*, 33(3), 804–818.

11. J. G. Mulle, W. G. Sharp, and J. F. Cubells (2013). "The Gut Microbiome: A New Frontier in Autism Research." *Current Psychiatry Reports*, 15(2): 337.

12. P. S. Lemer. (2019). *Outsmarting Autism: Build Healthy Foundations for Communication, Socialization, and Behavior at All Ages*, expanded and updated. Berkeley: North Atlantic Books, 331.

13. S. Porges (2017). *The Pocket Guide to the Polyvagal Theory: The Transformative Power of Feeling Safe*. New York: W. W. Norton.

14. C. Demopoulos, M. S. Arroyo, W. Dunn, Z. Strominger, E. H. Sherr, and E. Marco (2015). "Individuals with Agenesis of the Corpus Callosum Show Sensory Processing Differences as Measured by the Sensory Profile." *Neuropsychology*, 29(5): 751–58.

15. J. P. Owen, E. J. Marco, S. Desai, E. Fourie, J. Harris, S. S. Hill, A. B. Arnett, and P. Mukherjee (2013). "Abnormal White Matter Microstructure in Children with Sensory Processing Disorders." *NeuroImage: Clinical*, 2, 844–53.

16. T. Grandin (2008). *Thinking in Pictures: My Life with Autism*. New York: Knopf Doubleday, 69.

17. N. Levit-Binnun, M. Davidovitch, and Y. Golland (2013). "Sensory and Motor Secondary Symptoms as Indicators of Brain Vulnerability." *Journal of Neurodevelopmental Disorders*, 5(1), 1–21.

18. K. McMahon, D. Anand, M. Morris-Jones, and M. Z. Rosenthal (2019). "A Path from Childhood Sensory Processing Disorder to Anxiety Disorders: The Mediating Role of Emotion Dysregulation and Adult Sensory Processing Disorder Symptoms." *Frontiers in Integrative Neuroscience*, 13(22).

19. E. J. Marco, A. B. Aitken, V. P. Nair, et al. (2018). "Burden of De Novo Mutations and Inherited Rare Single Nucleotide Variants in

Children with Sensory Processing Dysfunction." *BMC Medical Genomics*, 11(50).

Chapter Four: Understanding Sensory Processing—and What Can Go Amiss

1. Mahler (2016). *Interoception*, 31.
2. C. Koscinski (2018). *Interoception: How I Feel: Sensing My World from the Inside Out*. Pocketbooks for Special Needs.
3. S. Herculano-Houzel (2012). "The Remarkable, Yet Not Extraordinary, Human Brain as a Scaled-Up Primate Brain and Its Associated Cost." *Proceedings of the National Academy of Sciences*, 109 (Supplement 1), 10661–68.
4. Ayres (2005). *Sensory Integration and the Child*, 28.
5. With permission of Anita C. Bundy and Jane Koomar, illustration adapted from chapter 11, "Orchestrating Intervention: The Art of Practice," in A. C. Bundy, S. J. Lane, and E. A. Murray, *Sensory Integration: Theory and Practice*, 2nd ed. (2002), 256. Philadelphia: F.A. Davis. The textbook's 3rd edition, by A. C. Bundy and S. J. Lane (2020), does not include the illustration.
6. Ayres (2005). *Sensory Integration and the Child*, 55.
7. Ayres (2005). *Sensory Integration and the Child*, 47.
8. B. Eide and F. Eide (2007). *The Mislabeled Child: Looking Beyond Behavior to Find the True Sources and Solutions for Children's Learning Challenges*. New York: Hachette, 310.
9. Jed Baker (2008). *No More Meltdowns*. Arlington, TX: Future Horizons, 5.
10. S. C. Wayland, parenting coach, Guiding Exceptional Parents, at www.guidingexceptionalparents.com (2021). Personal communication.
11. Ayres (1972). *Sensory Integration and Learning Disorders*. Los Angeles: Western Psychological Services, 134.
12. Ayres (2005). *Sensory Integration and the Child*, 87.

Chapter Five: How to Tell if Your Child Has SPD in the Tactile Sense

1. Ayres (1972). *Sensory Integration and Learning Disorders*, 61.

Chapter Six: How to Tell if Your Child Has SPD in the Vestibular Sense

1. Ayres (1972). *Sensory Integration and Learning Disorders*, 60.

2. Ayres (2005). *Sensory Integration and the Child*, 40.
3. Ayres (2005). *Sensory Integration and the Child*, 43.

Chapter Ten: Diagnosis and Treatment

1. Individuals with Disabilities Education Act, or IDEA 04 (2004). 20 U.S.C. § 1400.
2. Free appropriate public education for students with disabilities: requirements under section 504 of the Rehabilitation Act of 1973 (2010). Washington, DC: U.S. Department of Education, Office for Civil Rights.
3. Some assessment tools for children are: Sensory Integration and Praxis Tests (Ayres, 1989); Sensory Profile 2 (W. Dunn, 2014); Sensory Processing Measure-2 (L. D. Parham, C. L. Ecker, H. Miller-Kuhaneck, D. Henry, and T. Glennon, 2017); and the upcoming Sensory Processing Three Dimensions Scale (Miller, Schoen, Mulligan, unpublished).
4. *Diagnostic Classification of Mental Health and Developmental Disorders of Infancy and Early Childhood*, or DC:0-5 (2016). Washington, DC: Zero to Three.
5. V. Spielmann (2020). "The Interplay of Regulation, Relationships and Sensory Processing: Impact on Function and Participation." *Sensory Integration Education News*, SensorNet, 55: 24–26.
6. Ayres (2005). *Sensory Integration and the Child*, 17.

Chapter Eleven: Your Child at Home

1. J. J. Gibson (2014). "The Theory of Affordances (1979)." Chapter 9 in *The People, Place, and Space Reader*, edited by J. J. Gieseking, William Mangold, et al. London: Routledge.
2. T. A. May-Benson and S. A. Cermak (2007). "Development of an Assessment for Ideational Praxis." *American Journal of Occupational Therapy*, 61:2, 148–53.
3. Ayres and Cermak (2011). *Ayres Dyspraxia Monograph, 25th Anniversary Edition*. Torrance, CA: Pediatric Therapy Network, 67.

Chapter Thirteen: Coping with Your Child's Emotions

1. Shapiro, with S. Wayland. "The Gander" is at www.parentchild journey.com.
2. Floortime® approach, developed by S. Greenspan and S. Wieder (1980s). www.icdl.com/ and www.profectum.org.

Glossary

Academic learning: The development of conceptual skills, such as learning to read words and multiply numbers, and to apply what one learns today to what one learned yesterday.

Activity level: The degree of one's mental, emotional, or physical arousal. Activity level can be high, low, or in between.

Acuity: The keen perception of a sight, sound, or other sensation.

Adaptive behavior: The ability to respond actively and purposefully to changing circumstances and new sensory experiences.

Affordance: A quality about an object in the environment that invites a person's interaction. Affordances of a box are that it is fillable, closable, and pushable.

Arousal: A state of the nervous system ranging from sleep to awake, from low to high. The optimal state of arousal is the "just right" midpoint between boredom and anxiety, where we feel alert and calm.

Articulation: The production of speech sounds.

Attention deficit hyperactivity disorder (ADHD): An umbrella term for a problem interfering with one's ability to attend to and stay focused on meaningful tasks, control one's impulses, and regulate one's activity level. The main symptoms of this neurologically based disorder are hyperactivity, inattention (distractibility), and/or impulsivity.

Audition: The ability to receive and apprehend sounds; hearing.

Auditory discrimination: The ability to receive, identify, differentiate, understand, and respond to sounds. Discriminative functions include:

    Association—Relating novel sound to familiar sound.

    Attention—Maintaining focus sufficiently to listen to voices and sounds.

    Cohesion—Uniting various ideas into a coherent whole and drawing inferences from what is said.

    Discrimination—Differentiating among sounds.

    Figure-ground—Distinguishing between sounds in the foreground and the background.

Localization—Identifying the source of a sound.

Memory—Remembering what was said.

Sequencing—Putting what was heard in order.

Tracking—Following a sound as it moves.

Auditory training: A method of sound stimulation designed to improve a person's listening and communicative skills, learning capabilities, motor coordination, body awareness, and self-esteem.

Autism: A lifelong multisystem disability, usually appearing during the first three years of life, which severely impairs the person's sensory processing, verbal and nonverbal communication, social interaction, imagination, problem-solving, and development.

Autonomic nervous system: One of the three components of the nervous system; controls automatic, unconscious bodily functions, such as breathing, sweating, shivering, and digesting.

Aversive response: A feeling of revulsion and repugnance toward a sensation, accompanied by an intense desire to avoid or turn away from it.

Basic visual skills: Unconscious mechanisms of sight.

Behavior: Whatever one does, through actions, feelings, perceptions, thoughts, words, or movements, in response to stimulation.

Bilateral coordination: The ability to use both sides of the body together in a smooth and simultaneous manner.

Bilateral integration: The neurological process of integrating sensations from both sides of the body; the foundation for bilateral coordination.

Binocularity (binocular vision; eye teaming): The basic eye-motor skill of forming a single visual image from two images that the eyes separately record.

Body awareness, body percept, or body scheme: The mental picture of one's own body parts, where they are, how they interrelate, and how they move.

Body position: The placement of one's head, limbs, and trunk. Proprioception is the sense of body position.

Brain: The portion of the CNS that receives sensory messages; integrates, modulates, and organizes them; and sends out messages to produce motor, language, or emotional responses.

Brain behavior: Pertaining to the relationship of incoming sensory messages and outgoing motor, language, or emotional responses.

Central nervous system (CNS): The part of the nervous system, consisting of the brain and the spinal cord, that coordinates the activity of the entire nervous system.

Crossing the midline: Using a hand, foot, or eye on the opposite side of the body.

Defensive (or protective) system: The component of a sensory system that alerts one to real or potential danger and causes a self-protective response. This system is innate.

Defensiveness: The tendency to respond to certain harmless sensations as if they were dangerous or painful; overresponsivity.

Developmental delay: The acquisition of specific skills after the expected age. Early intervention may help the child catch up.

Developmental disability: A condition caused by an impairment in physical, learning, language, or behavior areas. It may begin in utero and continues as a child grows, impacting daily functioning and usually lasting throughout the person's life span.

Discrimination: The awareness of sensory input and the ability to distinguish its details within a particular sense.

Discriminative system: The component of a sensory system that allows one to distinguish differences among and between stimuli. This system is not innate but develops with time and practice.

Down syndrome: A congenital disorder, caused by an extra chromosome, which alters the typical development of the brain and body, resulting in intellectual disability and sensory processing challenges.

Dyscalculia: A learning disability related to grasping concepts of numbers, time, and space.

Dysgraphia: A learning disability in transcription, which involves handwriting, typing, and spelling.

Dyslexia: A learning disability involving severe difficulty in using or understanding language while listening, speaking, reading, writing, or spelling.

Dyspraxia: Difficulty in conceptualizing, motor planning, sequencing, and carrying out unfamiliar actions in a skillful manner. (See **Praxis**.)

Early intervention: Treatment or therapy to prevent problems or to improve a young child's health and development, such as eyeglasses or ear tubes for medical problems, and speech/language therapy or occupational therapy for developmental problems.

Emotional security: The sense that one is lovable and loved, that other people are trustworthy, and that one has the competence to function effectively in everyday life.

Enuresis: Involuntary urination in a child five years or older when no physical abnormality exists.

Essential fatty acids: Substances from fats that must be provided by foods because the body cannot make them and yet must have them for health.

Evaluation: The use of assessment tools, such as tests and observations, to measure a person's developmental level and individual skills, or to identify a possible difficulty.

Excitation: The neurological process of activating incoming sensory receptors to promote connections between sensory input and behavioral output.

Expressive language: The spoken or written words and phrases that one produces to communicate feelings and thoughts to others.

Extension: The pull of the muscles away from the front of the body; straightening or stretching.

External senses: The senses of touch, smell, taste, vision, and hearing; the environmental senses.

Extrasensory: Pertaining to extraordinary grace, artistry, or talent of many individuals with SPD.

Eye-hand coordination: The efficient teamwork of the eyes and hands, necessary for activities such as playing with toys, dressing, and writing.

Eye-motor skills: Movements of muscles in the eyes; also ocular-motor skills.

    Eye-hand coordination—The efficient teamwork of the eyes and hands.

    Fixation—Steady attention on an object.

    Focusing—Accommodating one's vision smoothly between near and distant objects.

    Saccades—Efficient movement of the eyes from point to point.

    Smooth pursuits (tracking)—Following a moving object or line of print with the eyes.

Fetal alcohol syndrome: A set of symptoms, including growth retardation, facial abnormalities, intellectual disability, and developmental delay, caused by the mother's chronic alcoholism during pregnancy.

Fight-or-flight response (or fight-flight-freeze-fright response): The instinctive reaction to defend oneself from real or perceived danger by becoming aggressive, withdrawing, or being unable to move.

Fine-motor: Referring to movement of the small muscles in the fingers, toes, eyes, and tongue.

Fixing: Pressing one's elbows into one's sides or one's knees together for more stability.

Flexion: Movement of the muscles around a joint to pull a body part toward its front or center; bending.

Floortime®: Intervention developed by Stanley I. Greenspan, MD, and Serena Wieder, PhD, that fosters children's healthy emotional development through intensive one-on-one interactions with adults on the child's level.

Fluctuating responsivity: A combination of overresponsivity and under-responsivity as the child's brain rapidly shifts back and forth.

Force: (See **Grading of movement**.)

Four Levels: Dr. Ayres's concept of the smooth, sequential development of sensory integration, from infancy through elementary school age.

Fragile X syndrome: A set of symptoms, including intellectual disability, facial anomalies, and deficits in communicative, behavioral, social, and motor skills; caused by an abnormality of the X chromosome.

Grading of movement (force): The ability to flex and extend muscles according to how much pressure is necessary to exert; a function of proprioception.

Gravitational insecurity: Extreme fear and anxiety that one will fall when one's head position changes or when moving through space, resulting from poor vestibular and proprioceptive processing.

Gross-motor: Referring to movement of large muscles in the arms, legs, and trunk.

Gustatory sense: The sense of perceiving flavor; taste.

Gut microbiome: All the microorganisms, bacteria, viruses, protozoa, fungi, and their genetic material that exist in the gastrointestinal tract. Communication between gut and brain via the vagus nerve is important for self-regulation, metabolism, immune system, emotions, etc. Disrupted gut-brain communication may be a contributing factor in SPD and autism.

Habituation: The neurological process of tuning out familiar sensations.

Hand preference: Right- or left-handedness, established as lateralization develops.

Hyperactivity: Excessive mobility, motor function, or activity, such as finger tapping, jumping from one's seat, or constantly moving some part of the body; "fidgetiness."

Hyperlexia: Unusually advanced reading ability and intense fascination with letters and numbers at a very young age, without reading comprehension and verbal communication skills.

Hyper-reactivity and **Hypo-reactivity:** Exaggerated neurological and physiological processes that we cannot observe and that may cause over- and underresponsive behavior.

Ideation: The process of forming or conceiving of a novel and complex action to take; the first step in praxis.

Impulse control: Difficulty in restraining one's actions, words, or emotions.

Increased tolerance for movement: Underresponsivity to typical amounts of movement stimulation; often characterized by craving for intense movement experiences such as rocking and spinning.

Individualized Education Program (IEP): A legal document specifying the needs of a child identified as having a disability and providing for special education and related services.

Individuals with Disabilities Education Act, P.L. 99-457, and amendments: (IDEA): This legislation requires school districts to provide occupational therapy as a related service to children who need it in order to benefit from education.

Inhibition: The neurological process that checks one's overreaction to sensations.

Inner drive: Every person's self-motivation to participate actively in experiences that promote sensory processing.

Inner ear: The organ that receives sensations of the pull of gravity and of changes in balance and head position.

Integration: The combination of many parts into a unified, harmonious whole.

Intellectual disability: Significant impairments in reasoning, learning, and problem-solving, and in adaptive behavior, originating before the age of twenty-two.

Internal eyes: Body awareness.

Internal senses: The subconscious interoceptive, vestibular, and proprioceptive senses that regulate bodily functions, such as heart rate, hunger, arousal, balance, and movement. Also called the somatosensory senses.

Interoception: The body-centered sense involving both the conscious awareness and the unconscious regulation of bodily processes of the heart, liver, stomach, and other internal organs.

Intersensory integration: The convergence of sensations of touch, body position, movement, sight, sound, and smell.

Intolerance to movement: The overreactivity to moving or being moved rapidly, often characterized by extreme distress when spinning or by avoidance of movement through space.

Kinesthesia: The conscious awareness of joint position and body movement in space, such as knowing where to place one's feet when climbing stairs, without visual cues.

Language: The organized use of words and phrases to interpret what one hears or reads and to communicate one's thoughts and feelings.

Lateralization: The process of establishing dominance of one side of the brain for directing skilled movement on the opposite side of the body, while the other side of the body is used for stabilization. Laterality is the preference of one's right or left hand, foot, or eye, e.g., right-handedness.

Learned helplessness: The tendency to depend on others for guidance and decisions, to lack self-help skills, and to be a passive learner; often related to poor self-esteem.

Learning disability: An identified difficulty with reading, writing, spelling, computing, and communicating. (SPD may cause significant learning problems that are often not recognized or identified as learning disabilities.)

Limbic system: The part of the brain that processes all sensory messages and is involved primarily with emotions and inner drive; the "seat of emotions"; the "smell brain."

Linear movement: A motion in which one moves in a line, from front to back, side to side, or up and down.

Low tone: (See **Muscle tone**.)

Meltdown: The process, usually caused by excessive sensory stimulation, of becoming "undone" or "unglued," accompanied by screaming, writhing, and deep sobbing.

Modulation: The brain's ability to regulate and organize the degree, intensity, and nature of the person's response to sensory input in a graded and adaptive manner.

Motor control: The ability to regulate and monitor the motions of one's muscles for coordinated movement.

Motor coordination: The ability of several muscles or muscle groups to work together harmoniously to perform movements.

Motor learning: The process of mastering simple movement skills essential for developing more complex movement skills.

Motor planning: The ability to organize and sequence the steps of an unfamiliar and complex body movement in a coordinated manner; a piece of praxis.

Muscle tone: The degree of tension normally present when one's muscles are relaxed, or in a resting state; a function of the vestibular system, enabling the person to maintain body position. **Low tone** is the lack of supportive muscle tone, usually with increased mobility at the joints; the person with low tone seems "loose and floppy."

Neurology: The science of the nerves and the nervous system. A neurologist is a physician who diagnoses and treats diseases of the brain and CNS, but usually not SPD.

Neuromuscular: Relating to the relationship of nerves and muscles.

Neuron: The nerve cell, which is the functional and structural unit of the nervous system and the fundamental building block of the brain. Sensory neurons receive messages from receptors in the eyes, ears, skin, muscles, joints, and organs, and motor neurons send out messages to the body for appropriate responses.

Occupational therapy (OT): The use of purposeful activity to maximize the health of an individual who is limited by a physical, cognitive, psychosocial, developmental, or adverse environmental condition. OT encompasses evaluation, assessment, treatment, and consultation. OT-SI includes therapy using play-based sensory-motor activities in a sensory integration framework. An occupational therapist (also OT) is a health professional trained in the biological, physical, medical, and behavioral sciences, including neurology, anatomy, development, kinesiology, orthopedics, psychiatry, and psychology.

Ocular-motor: (See **Eye-motor skills**.)

Olfactory sense: The sense that perceives odor; smell.

Optometrist or developmental optometrist: A specialist who examines eyes, prescribes lenses, and provides vision therapy to prevent or eliminate visual problems and enhance a person's visual performance.

Oral apraxia: A sensory-based motor problem affecting the ability to produce and sequence sounds necessary for speech.

Oral-motor skills: Movements of muscles in the mouth, lips, tongue, and jaw, including sucking, biting, crunching, chewing, and licking.

Oscillation: Up-and-down or to-and-fro linear movement, such as swinging, bouncing, and jumping.

Overresponsivity: Observable behavior involving a quick or intense response to sensory stimuli that others usually perceive as benign; characterized by exaggerated, negative, and emotional responses (fight-or-flight) or withdrawal (flight or freeze).

Passive movement: The act of being moved by something or someone.

Passive touch: The act of being touched by something or someone without initiating it.

Perception: The meaning that the brain gives to sensory input.

Perceptual-motor skill: The ability to receive, interpret, and use information from the senses and to integrate these sensations with movement to carry out voluntary physical actions. Some perceptual-motor skills are bilateral coordination, body awareness, crossing the midline, and laterality.

Peripheral nervous system (PNS): One of the three components of the nervous system. Through the spinal cord, peripheral nerves in one's skin, eyes, ears, muscles, and organs send sensory impulses to the brain and receive motor impulses from the brain.

Pervasive developmental disorder: Severe, overall impairment in the ability to regulate sensory experiences, affecting the child's affect and

behavior, interaction with others, and communication skills; similar
to, but milder than, autism.

Physical therapy: A health profession devoted to improving one's physical
abilities through activities that strengthen muscular control and motor coordination, especially of the large muscles.

Plasticity: The ability of the brain to change or to be changed as a result of
activity, especially as one responds to sensations.

Polyvagal theory: Stephen Porges's concept pertaining to the role of the
vagus cranial nerve in connecting messages between the heart, lungs,
and gut with the brain to regulate emotions, social relationships, and
fear response.

Postural background adjustments: Automatic movements in one's trunk
and limbs, allowing a person to use only the muscles necessary for a
particular motion.

Postural difference or challenge: Difficulty with moving or stabilizing the
body to meet the demands of the environment or a particular motor
task.

Postural stability: The feeling of security and self-confidence when moving in space, based on one's body awareness. SPD may cause postural
insecurity, the feeling that one's body is not stable.

Praxis: The ability to interact successfully with the physical environment;
to ideate, plan, organize, and carry out a sequence of unfamiliar actions; and to do what one needs and wants to do. The term denotes
voluntary and coordinated action. **Motor planning** is often used as a
synonym.

Prefrontal cortex: The cortical lobe in the brain that coordinates speech,
reasoning, remembering, problem-solving, self-control, and planning
ahead.

Problem feeding: The inability or refusal to eat certain foods, caused by
sensory processing difficulties, including visual and fine-motor challenges, and affecting nutritional and emotional development.

Proprioception/proprioceptive sense (the body position sense): The unconscious awareness of sensations coming from one's muscles, joints,
and ligaments that provides information about when and how muscles contract or stretch; when and how joints bend, extend, or are
pulled; and where each part of the body is and how it is moving.

Psychotherapy: Treatment by psychological means of mental, emotional,
or behavior problems.

Receptive language: The ability to understand how words express ideas
and feelings; language that one takes in by listening and reading.

Receptors: Special cells, located throughout one's body, that receive
specific sensory messages and send them for processing to the CNS.

Reflex: An automatic, innate response to sensory stimulation.

Regulatory disorder: A significant problem with adapting to changing conditions, such as self-calming when distressed, falling asleep and waking up, eating, digesting, eliminating, paying attention, participating socially, and processing sensations.

Reptilian brain: In evolutionary terms, the oldest part of the brain, controlling reflexive, instinctive behavior; the "primitive brain."

Rotary movement: Turning or spinning in circles.

Satiety: Fullness.

Screening: A quick, informal procedure for the early identification of children's health or developmental problems.

Selective mutism: A childhood anxiety disorder characterized by the inability to speak and communicate comfortably in select social settings.

Self-help skills: Competence in taking care of one's personal needs, such as bathing, dressing, eating, grooming, and studying.

Self-regulation: The ability to control one's activity level and state of alertness, as well as one's emotional, mental, or physical responses to sensations; self-organization.

Self-therapy: Active, voluntary participation in experiences that promote self-regulation, such as spinning in circles to stimulate one's vestibular system.

Sensitization: The process of interpreting stimuli as important, unfamiliar, or harmful, even if the stimuli are unimportant, familiar, and benign.

Sensory-based motor difference: A problem with movement, such as postural challenges and dyspraxia, resulting from inefficient sensory processing.

Sensory craving: The constant quest for excessive sensory stimulation.

Sensory discrimination difference: A problem in discerning the characteristics of stimuli and the differences among and between stimuli within one sensory system.

Sensory-enriched life: A planned and scheduled activity program that an occupational therapist develops to help a person become more self-regulated at home and at school.

Sensory integration (SI): The part of sensory processing whereby sensations from one or more sensory systems connect in the brain.

Sensory integration theory: A concept based on neurology, research, and behavior that explains the brain-behavior relationship.

Sensory integration treatment: A technique of occupational therapy that provides playful, meaningful activities that enhance an individual's sensory intake and lead to more adaptive functioning in daily life. The emphasis is on improving sensory-motor processing and on "flourishing," rather than on skill training.

Sensory-enriched life: An individualized sensory-motor activity program (sometimes called a "sensory diet") developed by an OT to meet the physical and emotional needs of a specific child's nervous system. The purpose is to help the child become better regulated and more focused, adaptable, and skillful, at home and at school.

Sensory modulation difference: A problem with regulating and organizing the degree, intensity, and nature of responses to sensory input in a graded and adaptive manner.

Sensory-motor: Pertaining to the brain-behavior process of taking in sensory messages and reacting with a physical response.

Sensory processing difference/disorder (SPD): Difficulty in the way the brain takes in, integrates, organizes, and uses sensory information, causing a person to have problems interacting effectively in the everyday environment. Sensory stimulation may cause difficulty in one's movement, emotions, attention, relationships, or adaptive responses.

Sensory processing machine: Dr. A. Jean Ayres's term for the brain.

Sequencing: Putting movements, sounds, sights, objects, thoughts, letters, and numbers in consecutive order, according to time and space.

Social pragmatics: The use of language and gestures to interact with others, such as when greeting them, telling them things, and making requests and demands.

Social skills: Effective interaction and communication with others, necessary for developing and keeping friendships. Social pragmatic skills are the ability to use spoken language and nonverbal gestures to interact successfully with others.

Somatosensory: Referring to tactile-proprioceptive discrimination of touch sensations and body position; body sensing.

Special education: Individualized instruction for the child who has difficulty learning at school.

Specialization: The process whereby one part of the brain becomes most efficient at a particular function.

Speech: The physical act of communicating a verbal message.

Speech-and-language therapy: Treatment to help a person develop or improve articulation, communication skills (social pragmatics), and oral-motor skills, including eating.

Spinal cord: The long, thick cord of nervous tissue that receives tactile and proprioceptive messages from skin, joints, and muscles, and that sends out motor messages for movement.

Splinter skill: An isolated ability that one develops with much effort, but that one cannot generalize for other purposes.

State: The degree of one's attentiveness, mood, or motor response to sensory stimulation.

Stereotypical behavior: Nonproductive, repetitive, and habitual actions often associated with autism.

Stimulus (pl., stimuli): Something that activates a sensory receptor and produces a response.

Syndrome: A group of unrelated, co-occurring characteristics, varying in severity from one individual to another, such as cognitive impairment and small ears, hands, and feet in a person with Down syndrome.

Tactile discrimination: The awareness of touching or of being touched by something; the ability to distinguish differences in touch sensations; and the awareness of the physical attributes of an object, such as its size, shape, temperature, density, and texture.

Tactile-proprioceptive: Referring to simultaneous sensations of touch and body position.

Tactile sense (the sense of touch): The sensory system that receives sensations of pressure, vibration, movement, temperature, and pain, primarily through receptors in the skin and hair. Defensive receptors respond to light or unexpected touch and help a person avoid bodily harm; discriminative receptors provide information about the tactile qualities of the object or person being touched.

Touch pressure: The tactile stimulus that causes receptors in the skin to respond.

Active touch is using one's hands, feet, and mouth to gather tactile information about objects in the environment.

Deep pressure, such as a hug, activates receptors in the discriminative system.

Light touch, such as a kiss, activates receptors in the protective system.

Passive touch is being touched by something or someone.

Tourette syndrome: A neurological condition involving repetitive, involuntary movements and vocalizations (tics).

Triune brain: Paul MacLean's theory that the brain is composed of three systems (the reptilian complex, the limbic system, and the cerebrum).

Twice-exceptional (2e): Referring to children who are gifted in some ways and challenged in others, e.g., intellectually talented students with learning disabilities or sensory-motor difficulties.

Underconnectivity theory: Reduced anatomical and functional connections between front and back areas of the brain, affecting sensory processing, language, executive thinking, relationships, etc.

Underresponsivity: Undersensitivity to sensory stimuli, characterized by a tendency to be unaware of sensations or to withdraw and be difficult to engage; a subtype of sensory modulation differences.

Unilateral coordination: Smooth, independent use of one side of the body, necessary for writing and handling tools.

Vestibular-proprioceptive: Referring to simultaneous sensations of head and body position when one moves.

Vestibular sense (the balance and movement sense): The sensory system that responds to the pull of gravity, providing information about the head's position in relation to the surface of the earth, and coordinating movements of the eyes, head, and body that affect equilibrium, muscle tone, vision, hearing, and emotional security. Receptors are in the inner ear.

Vision: The process of identifying sights, understanding what the eyes see, and preparing for a response.

Vision therapy: Treatment to help a person improve visual skills and to prevent learning-related visual problems; optometric visual training.

Visualization: The act of forming mental images of objects, people, or scenarios.

Visual discrimination: The ability to perceive and interpret sensory information received through the eyes and body as one interacts with the environment and moves one's body through space.

> **Attention**—The use of the eyes, brain, and body together long enough to stay with an activity.
>
> **Depth perception**—The ability to see objects in three dimensions and to judge relative distances between objects, or between oneself and objects.
>
> **Discrimination**—Discernment of likenesses and differences in size, shape, pattern, form, position, and color.
>
> **Figure-ground**—Differentiation between objects in the foreground and background.
>
> **Form constancy**—Recognition of a shape regardless of its size, position, or texture.
>
> **Memory**—Recognizing, associating, storing, and retrieving visual details.
>
> **Peripheral vision**—Awareness of images through the sides of the eyes.
>
> **Position in space**—Awareness of the spatial orientation of letters, words, numbers, or drawings on a page, or of an object in the environment.
>
> **Sequential memory**—Perception of words and pictures in order.

Spatial relationships—Awareness of directionality (how close objects are) and laterality (right/left, front/back, up/down), and how to move around objects.

Stable visual field—Discernment of which objects move and which stay still.

Visual-sensory integration—Combining sights with touch, movement, and other sensory messages.

Visualization—Forming and manipulating images of objects, people, or scenes in one's mind's eye.

Visual-motor skills: One's movements based on the discrimination of visual information.

Eye-ear coordination—The ability to see a letter or word, and say or use it.

Eye-foot coordination—The eyes' guidance of gross-motor activities.

Eye-hand coordination—The eyes' guidance of fine-motor tasks.

INDEX

Note: In this index, the word "differences" stands for "difficulties," "disorder," and "dysfunction." (See "A Word About Words," page xxv.)

Page numbers in *italics* refer to illustrations.

MacLean, Paul D., MD, 331
Mahler, Kelly, OTD, 25
Marco, Elysa, MD, 56
Martial arts, 363
May-Benson, Teresa A., ScD, 271
Mental health issues overlapping
    with SPD, xviii, 57–58, 230
Miller, Lucy Jane, PhD, xi, xxvi,
    12, 51
The Mislabeled Child (Eide and
    Eide), 87
Misophonia, 30, 61
Modulation. *See* Sensory
    modulation
Motor planning (part of Praxis).
    See also Sensory-based motor
    skills/differences
    activities to improve, 258,
        274, 278
    and auditory sense, 206,
        210, 216
    differences with, 16, 24, 93–94
    and proprioceptive sense, 165,
        174–75
    and tactile sense, 103–4, 113–14
    typically developing, 77, 82, 343
    and vestibular sense, 142, 152,
        159, 238, 274
Movement/Motor control/Motor
    coordination
    active and passive, 216
    activities to improve,
        278–80
    and auditory sense, 206–11,
        216–17, 221
    as basis of learning, 13
    charts/checklists, 12, 17, 20,
        23–25
    craving for movement, 8–9
        (Sebastian), 90
    development of, 82, 333,
        342–44

dyspraxia/postural issues, 12,
    22–25, 92–94
gravitational insecurity,
    142–43, 155
intolerance to movement, 86,
    134, 140–41, 154
and learning disabilities, 45–47
and proprioceptive sense, 160
    ff., 210
responses to linear and
    rotary movement, 138–39,
    141, 145
and self-regulation issues
    (eating/sleeping/toileting),
    29, 30–31, 33, 35
and smooth sensory processing,
    63, 69, 76–83, 334, 341–43
and speech, 28, 210
and tactile sense, 102, 113–16,
    130–31, 210
treatments for, 47, 153, 216,
    253, 256–61, 295
and vestibular sense, 5–6, 132
    ff., 142, 164, 210
and visual sense, 93, 139–40,
    183–203, 342
Muscle control/Muscle tone
    and auditory sense, 211
    checklists, 17, 20, 23
    and eating, 30–31
    and postural differences, 92
    and proprioceptive sense, 176,
        334, 342
    and tactile sense, 114
    treatments for differences with,
        258–59, 261–62
    typically developing, 76, 135,
        334, 342
    and vestibular sense, 135,
        148–49, 156–57,
        238–39
    and visual sense, 185

About the Author

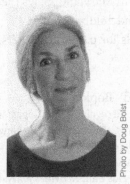

Photo by Doug Bolst

Carol Stock Kranowitz observed many children with sensory processing differences (SPD) and mild autism during her twenty-five-year career as a preschool teacher. To help them become more competent in their work and play, she studied sensory processing and sensory integration (SI) theory. She learned to help identify her young students' needs and to steer them into early intervention. Today, she speaks internationally about SPD's effect on children's learning and behavior and how families, teachers, therapists, and other professionals can support children as they grow.

Since its publication in 1998, the first book in her *Sync* series, *The Out-of-Sync Child*, has become one of the most popular books about sensory processing and related issues. It has been translated into sixteen languages and has sold one million copies.

A graduate of Barnard College of Columbia University, Carol has a master's degree in education and human development from The George Washington University. She is an advisory board member of STAR Institute for Sensory Processing in Colorado. She lives in Maryland, plays the cello, and dotes on five sensational grandchildren.

Carol's materials for parents, teachers, professionals, and children include:

"Out-of-Sync Child" Books

The Out-of-Sync Child: Recognizing and Coping with Sensory Processing Differences, third ed. (2022). New York: TarcherPerigee. Also available in an audio version (2016). New York: Random House.

The Out-of-Sync Child Has Fun: Activities for Kids with SPD, second ed. (2006). Perigee.

The Out-of-Sync Child Grows Up: Coping with Sensory Processing Disorder in the Adolescent and Young Adult Years (2016). TarcherPerigee.

Children's Books

The Goodenoughs Get in Sync: 5 Family Members Overcome Their Special Sensory Issues, rev. ed. (2019). Arlington, TX: Sensory World.

Absolutely No Dogs Allowed! (2015). Alphabet book by Asher Kranowitz, with Carol's guidelines for discussing senses and emotions with children. Sensory World.

101 Activities for Kids in Tight Spaces (1995). New York: St. Martin's.

Screening Manuals for Teachers and Therapists

Preschool SENsory Scan for Educators, or *Preschool SENSE* (2006). Arlington, TX: Sensory Resources.

Balzer-Martin Preschool Screening Program, with Lynn Balzer-
    Martin (1987). Washington, DC: St. Columba's Nursery School.
    www.stcolumbasnurseryschool.org.
Answers to Questions Teachers Ask About Sensory Integration, 3rd ed.,
    with Jane Koomar, Stacey Szklut, et al. (2014). Sensory World.

"In-Sync Child" Publications with Joye Newman

*Growing an In-Sync Child: Simple, Fun Activities to Help Every Child
    Develop, Learn and Grow* (2010). Perigee.
*In-Sync Activity Cards: 50 Simple, New Activities to Help Children
    Develop, Learn, and Grow* (2012). Sensory World. Also pub-
    lished as *The In-Sync Activity Card Book* (2015), Sensory World;
    and in digital format in English, French, Greek, Italian, and
    Spanish (2021). Greece: www.upbility.net.
The In-Sync Child Method webinars (2021). Ten-part series about
    child development and fun activities. In English at https://
    in-sync-child.com/the-in-sync-child-webinar-series/. In Greek
    at www.upbility.net.
A Year of Mini-Moves for the In-Sync Child (2021). Weekly schedules
    in digital format, in English, French, Greek, Italian, and
    Spanish, www.upbility.net); and in spiral-bound format in
    English, www.SensoryWorld.com (2022).

To learn about translations and other materials, visit www
.out-of-sync-child.com and www.insyncchild.com.

Also from

Carol Kranowitz

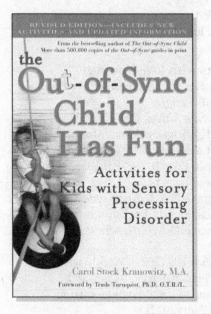

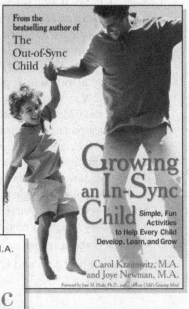